The Adventure of Birth

EXPERIENCES IN THE LAMAZE METHOD

OF PREPARED CHILDBIRTH

━━━━━━━━━━━━━━━━━━━━━━━

EDITED BY

Elisabeth D. Bing

SIMON AND SCHUSTER

NEW YORK

First printing

SBN 671-20486-6
Library of Congress Catalog Card Number: 75-101866
Manufactured in the United States of America
by The Book Press, Brattleboro, Vt.

1519722

Bunny was in the woods,
It was night.
It was cold and windy.

She had a funny feeling.
Little babies inside her—ready
To pop out from her body.

She started to cry
Because she was happy.

Then four baby bunnies
Came out of her body.
She kissed each one
As they came out.

—SIX-YEAR-OLD

Introduction

The telephone rings. My husband picks it up.

"Hello . . ." His voice always seems to be about an octave lower on the phone than in ordinary conversation. A man's voice at the other end of the phone says, "Hello there, I am one of Mrs. Bing's husbands," and I hear my husband answer, "So am I!" "Is Mrs. Bing in?" questions the voice on the other end. "I have to report that we have just had a baby, it's beautiful, and we are so happy. . . ."

And another phone call not long ago. This time I answered it.

"Mrs. Bing, Mrs. Bing," a man's voice says excitedly, "our membranes have broken, we are at the hospital, no contractions yet, everything under control! And what do you think? Evelyn is having her hair done there to look beautiful for our baby, and we are so excited!" I give a few last-minute instructions, encouragement, and a big hurray! for the baby which will be coming so soon. "O.K., Coach Bing," says the voice on the phone. "O.K., Coach Bing, we won't forget."

"We've just had a lovely little boy a half hour ago," says another man's voice over the phone, "and let me tell you what happened. . . ." And here followed a blow-by-blow description of the labor. "And when we started to push . . ."

I have been an instructor of "prepared childbirth" for many years. It is the psychoprophylactic method of childbirth, or Lamaze technique, which I have taught to several thousand young parents, an education technique that has been widely accepted in many parts of the United States and, of course, also in many countries all over the world.

After so many years of teaching, of holding workshops, of giving talks to professional groups, I feel it is time now that we let the young couples talk who have trained for the birth of their child, and to listen to their impressions, their feelings of happiness or uneasiness, or even their misgivings, about their venture into parenthood. The medical profession has written about prepared childbirth from its point of view, the nurses have often voiced their impressions, teachers of the psychoprophylactic method have published articles on teaching techniques. But in this little volume I would like to give the floor to our young parents, to hear from them how our training has affected them and perhaps to share their experiences with them.

Those of us who have been in this field of education have heard over and over again that it is the "neurotic woman" who wants to take a course in preparation for childbirth. I am afraid this accusation will have to be scrapped now. There simply are too many young parents demanding to participate in the birth of their children, and surely there can't be that many neurotics around all the time! We have been told that we create feelings of failure when circumstances do not permit a woman to fully participate when she gives birth, that women feel let down, frustrated or even ashamed if they need the good help of their physicians.

I grant you this may be true of a few isolated cases. However, anybody who takes the trouble to find out what our aims are and what we actually teach will soon realize that we never hold out "the method" as a panacea, as the only answer to having a good and healthy experience in labor. We prepare young parents for a difficult physical and emotional experience, we encourage learning and disciplined training, and we see the young husband in the role of his wife's coach. He supports her during labor, he encourages her, he gives her his strength and love, he is the rock she can lean on.

Not long ago I was explaining the Lamaze technique and the role of the husband in labor and delivery to a group of obstetricians. One physician remarked at the end that in his experience he had found that the young wife became emotionally too dependent on her husband during labor and delivery. My answer came before I could think: "I can't think of any other person in the world for a young wife to become emotionally dependent upon!"

It is my very strong conviction that a healthy family is one in which the husband is dominant, and I know that this has been found to be the case in all the many studies that have been made of family relations. It is the essence of marriage that a couple shares their life, that they not only experience everyday occurrences together but that they especially share and support each other in really important events in their life. I can't imagine many more important times in a marriage than giving birth to one's child. Surely it should be the husband's privilege, or, in fact, even his right, to be with his wife during the birth of their baby, if he so wants to. I absolutely agree with Dr. John Miller, who once called it a matter of "human rights" for the husband to attend the birth of his child.

It is not so long ago that almost all women delivered their babies in their homes, and the physician or the mid-

9

wife came to the young couple's home to help during the birth of the baby. I wonder if it would have occurred to the doctor or the midwife then to tell the husband to leave his own home and get out of the way? In fact, the doctor or midwife were guests in the couple's home: they were called in to assist and supervise, not to interfere. And I am sure they respected the family's dignity and way of life, and acted accordingly.

I am not in favor of home deliveries at all, but I feel strongly that we have lost a great deal of dignity and human approach in our endeavor to make childbirth safe for mother and child. Our aim is to bring the home into the hospital, and to recapture the excitement and warmth that could be—and should be—part of giving birth. And we should remember that every woman feels she is the center of the universe when she gives birth to her child. Her husband is part of this center of her universe, and he should be given an opportunity to fulfill this part.

Without sounding sentimental, I am convinced that such a shared experience makes a marriage into a very real and deeply felt partnership. The husband is not left out to see his baby only after birth, through a glass window. He has actually helped in the birth of his child, seen it and heard it take its first breath, and held it in his arms only a few minutes after birth. He can immediately relate to his child, and he shares with his wife the wonderful feeling of a great achievement.

It is comparatively easy to gather statistics and show from a medical point of view the advantages of prepared childbirth, and this has been done, and is still being done, in a number of studies. Psychologists and sociologists have studied young parents who have participated in the birth of their children, and excellent papers have been published on their findings.

In the following pages I am not concerned with evaluating results from the medical point of view or with making a study in depth from the psychological or sociological angle; I want to let the parents who were kind enough to allow me to use their letters speak for themselves, and let you make up your mind what you think about it all.

"O.K., Coach Bing . . . "

Jeremy

●●

DEAR MRS. BING:

I started to feel something Friday evening, December
20—not even real contractions, more like mild cramps.
Since it was four days before the baby's due date, and I
had seen the doctor that morning and he had said it
wouldn't be for a while, I ignored them and we had dinner and went to a movie. After we got home I checked
the time and found the cramps were coming around every
fifteen minutes—but still thought it was nothing.

I went to sleep with no trouble around 1 A.M. and slept
very soundly, but I woke up around 6:30 A.M. with a
contraction, still quite mild. I went to the bathroom and
found some mucus and blood, but then I had been having that for a couple of weeks previously and the doctor
had assured me it was nothing.

I went back to bed and back to sleep. However, this
time they were waking me up every ten to fifteen minutes.
My husband got up and fixed me some tea and I stayed
in bed reading stories to our daughter. Around 10 A.M.
Gerry suggested we call the doctor and just tell him what
was going on. We did, and he said to time them more
closely and call him back around 11:30—also that I should
make whatever provisions necessary for Leslie's care. Once

he said that, I felt for the first time that maybe it was the real thing.

I got up, dressed Leslie, made beds and generally straightened up. There wasn't much change in intensity, but the contractions were still coming, so I called the doctor back and he said to come to his office in about an hour and be ready to go to the hospital from there.

Gerry took Leslie and the dog over to our friend's house; meanwhile I was still quite sure we would be back to pick her up that afternoon. Naturally we had trouble getting a cab and arrived at the doctor's office shortly after 1 P.M. He looked out when we came in and said, "You look too comfortable to be in labor." I was meanwhile feeling rather foolish, convinced it was a false alarm and I was getting everyone excited for nothing. I must have had some premonition, however, because the night before I had insisted Gerry reread "Six Practical Lessons for an Easier Childbirth" before he went to sleep.

The doctor checked me and said, "You're ready, go right to the hospital. I'll meet you there in a few minutes." I was really surprised and suddenly very excited.

In the cab on the way to the hospital I did some slow breathing, not so much because I needed to—more for practice.

We arrived at the hospital around 2 P.M.—naturally at the wrong entrance, where everyone looked very startled and said, "Are you really in labor?" Whereupon they produced a wheelchair and gave me a ride to the labor room.

Gerry was right with me. The nurse pushing the chair told Gerry to go to a waiting room. He said no, he was going to be with me, and no one made any further protest. The nurse came in and said, "Oh, you're doing La-

14

maze. How wonderful! I want to have my babies the same way."

I undressed and the doctor stuck his head in to tell us he had arrived, and he gave Gerry a white coat to wear over his street clothes. The doctor ordered a partial prep and a low enema. Both experiences were uncomfortable when my first baby was born, because I was unprepared. Now I was expecting these procedures and easily took them in my stride.

Gerry and I sat around and joked and chatted. I did some slow breathing while he timed the contractions, which were now about five to seven minutes apart. The doctor examined me and said I was 4 cm dilated and everything was going quickly and well.

They started a drip of glucose and water, which wasn't as uncomfortable as I thought it would be. In fact, the glucose kept up my strength and prevented me from becoming dehydrated.

All the attendants understood I was doing Lamaze and waited very patiently until I was finished with a contraction before either listening for the baby's heartbeat or asking any questions.

The doctor checked me again and the baby had not dropped at all. At this point he started a drip, pitocin, a hormone that speeds up labor and increases the speed and effectiveness of the uterine contractions. He also ruptured the membranes. The contractions now started coming quite hard and fast, two to three minutes apart. At one point I shifted in the middle of a contraction from the slow breathing to the panting. I had used the slow breathing very comfortably for a long time but suddenly couldn't use it any more.

Gerry meanwhile was very busy popping lollipops in and

out of my mouth, wiping my brow, timing the contractions, keeping an eye on my relaxation and calling out the time of the contraction.

At about 4 P.M. the doctor examined me and said there was a good chance the baby would be born within the hour. Gerry and I got so excited (I had been in labor with the first baby for about twelve hours). The doctor, by the way, was absolutely marvelous; he was there the entire time, cheerful, understanding and informative.

Then things started to go much more slowly and I started to feel very nauseous (did not throw up, however). I got very, very sleepy. I dozed off between contractions, and when they started again I was having trouble waking up in time to keep on top of them.

Gerry kept putting cold water on my face, arms and feet, meanwhile saying very firmly, "Wake up . . . pant . . . keep going . . . deep breath . . . relax." The doctor examined me again and said I was 6 cm, at which point I got very discouraged. I thought I wasn't even near transition yet.

Gerry said he was going to step out and call to see how our daughter was getting on, but I really didn't want him to leave. Then, with the next contraction, I felt some rectal pressure, not a great deal, but I mentioned it to Gerry and the doctor. The doctor stepped out for a moment and then everything went crazy. With the next contraction I had tremendous pressure and an urge to push. I started blowing like crazy and yelled to Gerry in between blows to get the doctor. He was so startled that for a minute he didn't understand. Meanwhile I was blowing like a steam engine and I said, "Get him *fast!*"

Gerry ran out into the hall and yelled for the doctor, who came running, took one look at me and said, "Deliv-

16

ery room, *now!*" I was quickly helped onto a stretcher with wheels. The doctor threw Gerry white slippers, mask and hat, and we went careening down the hall, with me still blowing and Gerry and the doctor hopping along trying to keep up and get their equipment on.

I said, "Can I push?" and the doctor said, "Not yet." Gerry said, "Pant . . . blow . . . keep going." They rolled me onto the delivery table (which at this hospital has a tilted back, nice hand grips and a good mirror). The doctor said, "Keep blowing." They draped me quickly. Gerry asked if the baby had crowned yet, and the intern said no.

And then the doctor said, "The baby will be born with the next contraction. You can push." It came immediately. At some point he did an episiotomy, but I don't know when. Gerry held my head, I raised up, pushed once, and the doctor said, "Look." We looked, and there was the baby's head. "Don't push," he said. And suddenly there he was—all of him with one contraction. The doctor said, "It's a boy," held him up—and little Jeremy promptly peed all over me.

He was perfect, and in one second pink and kicking like crazy. Gerry and I were shouting and laughing and Jeremy was yelling. The doctor laid him on my belly and we admired our beautiful new son.

One more contraction and push—and the placenta was out. It was 6:30 P.M.

In general I had a very easy time, felt very comfortable —had no back labor at all. The slow breathing, the panting, worked perfectly.

The only rough time was, as I mentioned before, when I got sleepy. Also at that point my contractions were lasting much longer than sixty seconds and they seemed to run together. However, it never occurred to us that it was transition since the doctor had said I was only 6 cm dilated. So I never used the rhythmic transition breathing. But I sure did a lot of blowing and, as I said before, only two pushes—one for the baby and one for the placenta.

Gerry was a wonderful coach. For us to be able to share in the birth of our son was truly the ultimate experience.

Sincerely,
SHARON F.

THE HUSBAND'S EXPERIENCE

DEAR MRS. BING:

Anxiety: The fuel strike hit us the week before Sharon gave birth. Our building was totally without heat. We warmed ourselves before the oven in our kitchen. We went to bed looking like bulky bears in our four layers of sweaters. And Sharon was due any day. How could we bring a newborn baby back to a freezing apartment? How was our four-year-old daughter Leslie going to react to a baby brother or sister? Where were we going to find someone sensitive and competent with the new baby during the early weeks? And how was the birth going to go?

Sharon was getting bored with her big belly. She was at the stage where she was getting food stains on her clothing, as if this immense protuberance wasn't really part of her. Her attitude was: Come on, Baby, hurry up! But we were both very anxious. Not about the birth itself. The fuel strike, the change in our lives, the planning. We were beginning to snap at each other.

At Last: On the day Sharon's labor began I was wearing long red underwear, heavy boots, a plaid shirt, a bulky wool sweater and wool trousers. I had been sleeping in this

18

clothing for three nights. I was unshaven. I have no idea why I was so raunchy. Maybe I was dressed for a primitive frontier experience. The result was I began to sweat the moment we entered the hospital. I was unused to heated rooms. As the labor progressed, clothing came off me like leaves from an artichoke.

Labor: The labor room had all the charm of a labor union meeting hall. Harsh lighting, flaking walls, dreary institutional colors. But it felt great to be there. The nurses, the doctor, everyone seemed to be in tune with prepared childbirth. There wasn't any of that stupidity which we had encountered at another hospital where Sharon had our first child using the Lamaze method. The only disturbing thing was the weeping and shouting we heard from other women on the floor. I knew it was disturbing Sharon, but there was nothing to be done about it. It was like seeing a wrecked car full of bloody bodies the first time you drive a car.

Sharon started with deep breathing during contractions. I was busy timing and popping lollipops into her mouth. We were both elated. There was a sense of being absolutely alone together, a sort of true sexual intimacy. And Sharon looked beautiful, her face full of delicious color. Even the hospital gown looked good. And we were warm. Soon we hardly noticed the moans of the other women on the floor.

Second Stage: The contractions began to get closer together and to become more intense. Sharon began panting. The doctor examined her and said that she would probably give birth within an hour. We were both delighted. More panting. More timing. More licks on the lollipop. Sharon was thirsty. I wet a washcloth and she chewed on it. Sharon was getting sleepy. I wet her face with cold water. The doctor examined her again. He was disappointed.

Little further dilation. He said his estimate was wrong. It might be a long labor. "But," he added, "one never knows." Things could change immediately. I didn't know what to do. I wanted to call our friends. They had taken Leslie, our daughter, for the day. I wanted to talk to her. I didn't want her to feel deserted. But Sharon didn't want me to leave the room. She was getting more and more sleepy. She was still panting but it was difficult for her to concentrate. I was worried. If she couldn't concentrate now, what was going to happen when she went into transition? I bustled around, talked in a loud voice, put cold water on her face. I said, "Concentrate, concentrate, you'll lose control." Sharon replied in a sleepy voice, "I've lost control." I was shouting at her, "Nonsense, come, come on." Suddenly she started to blow very intensely. What the hell was going on? She wasn't in transition yet. Then she said in a surprisingly calm way, "Call the doctor." I thought she wanted to ask him a question. Then she said, "Yell for him, out in the hall." I finally woke up. I bellowed. The doctor came running. Sharon was still blowing like mad. The doctor examined her. "Into the delivery room," he shouted. He tossed me surgical clothes and slippers. Off we went down the hall, Sharon on a wheel table, blowing like a baby whale. I was struggling with my slippers as we ran.

Finale: In the delivery room I was poised behind Sharon to help her push. Finally the doctor said, "Push!" I had remembered to prop Sharon up with pillows and shoved at her back. The doctor said, "Here it comes!" And I looked. There was the back of the baby's head coming out of Sharon. And then a face. My face. The baby was turned around. I saw a penis come out, testicles. "A boy! A boy!" we shouted. We laughed, we cried. The doctor cut the umbilical cord. A nurse cleaned up my son and rested him on a table. My son had greeted the world by peeing on his mother.

The doctor pressed down on Sharon's belly to help her express the placenta. Then he began to examine her internally. She was in pain and gripped my hand. I was worried. Was anything wrong? He said that everything was all right.

They left us alone for a time. We looked at our son. He was so beautiful. I felt a sense of ecstasy. And a love and warmth for Sharon that was thick and palpable and alive. In my head I kept seeing the birth, the body of my son emerging from Sharon's body. I didn't want to lose that image ever. The colors. His crying. Sharon's sounds of joy. We kissed and kissed again and looked at our son. What a woman, what a woman she is, I thought. And she is my wife and she loves me.

Epilogue: The fuel strike was settled and little Jeremy, weighing seven pounds, came home to a warm apartment. A Swedish girl who had worked for us a year before was there to help Sharon during the early weeks. Leslie loves her little brother and doesn't seem to be wrecked by any sibling distresses. And I, besides witnessing the dramatic, majestic birth of my son, love Sharon more than ever. Maybe the experience has confirmed in both of us our feelings about what a woman is: Not an object. Not a sexual joy, but a sexual partner. Not a frail, fey little thing deserving of sentimental tenderness laced with condescension. But a woman. Brave, enduring, strong, gentle, life-giving and life-enhancing. One who owns her own mind and her own body. And who gives of that body and that mind generously.

Sincerely,
GERRY F.

Timothy

●●●

DEAR MRS. BING:

On August 15 at 5:30 P.M.—two weeks past my due
date—I wearily reported to my doctor's office for a checkup.
A full week before that he had assured me the cervix was
softening nicely; however, it was my secret belief that the
whole thing was a hoax and that I was fated to drag
through life, huge belly and all.

This visit was different. My doctor said I was in the
early stages of labor—indeed, I was dilated 2 cm—and he
really brought me down to earth when he announced,
"Your baby will be born tomorrow, August sixteenth."
I scarcely remember the long bus ride home. My husband
and I had a gin and tonic to celebrate and I prepared his
dinner (I had been told to skip mine), still feeling no
contractions.

My doctor called at 11 P.M., and since I had very little
progress to report he told me to have a light snack and try
and get some sleep. However, I was far beyond sleeping,
and when my brother-in-law and sister-in-law and a friend
dropped in we decided to play poker. I am perhaps the
world's worst poker player, although fascinated by the game.
Shortly after the game started I began to notice faint contractions and would hold up a hand and yell "Time!" at
which point the men would go for their watches and some-

22

one would jot down the time. The contractions were coming every seven to eight minutes, slowly increasing in intensity, and I was winning at poker. (I would like to offer a fast game of poker as a substitute for the first Lamaze breathing exercises—however, it is essential that you win at the game; otherwise this substitute method won't work!)

I was a little self-conscious about doing the breathing exercise in front of our guests but I did relax completely with each contraction and breathed slowly.

After the contractions had been coming every five minutes for an hour and a half, I telephoned my doctor and was told to come on in to the hospital.

It was 5:30 A.M. when I arrived in the labor room of the hospital. My doctor was there to greet me, and shortly after I was prepped he examined me and said I was 3 cm dilated. He then broke the membrane. Almost immediately the contractions became stronger and closer together. I found that I had to go directly into accelerated breathing, and I also soon discovered that the massage of my abdomen was doing little if any good—I was having back labor. I was sitting up in bed at this point and found that rolling my fists in the small of my back helped tremendously. Sometimes my husband would do it for me,—but generally I found that I was better able to do it myself.

I tried the side and kneeling positions to ease the back labor but with little success. I found it very difficult to do the accelerated breathing in the kneeling position and therefore was happier in the old familiar sitting position with my fists in my back. (Maybe I should have varied my positions in practice more.)

At 6:30 A.M. my doctor examined me and said I was 5 cm dilated. I was thrilled at the progress I had made in

23

an hour and at the fact that I was halfway home. The contractions were now coming every two to three minutes and quite strong.

My husband was a tremendous help—I could never have made it without him. He timed every contraction, and at the peak of each one, when I'd get a faint touch of nausea and really have to dig my fists in my back to ease that situation, I knew that if I just hung on until Steve said "Forty-five seconds," the worst would be over and another contraction would be behind me. I also discovered that the sooner I started my accelerated breathing just prior to the start of a contraction, and the more involved I got in the mechanics of the exercise, the less I felt the contraction. I found thinking about riding the wave helpful.

My doctor left instructions for me to have Demerol if I needed it, and occasionally, if I'd gotten off to a bad start with a contraction, I would think about the dear old Demerol. However, I was very drowsy at this point, and Steve mopped my face with a cold sponge whenever I showed signs of nodding. Around 9 A.M., in the midst of a contraction, I was startled by a sudden urge to push. After a few confused seconds, I started blowing out. Shortly after the contraction ended the resident came in and Steve told him I thought the urge to push had begun. After an examination, the resident announced I was 7 cm and obviously going into transition. The contractions were often quite close together, sometimes lasting as long as seventy-five seconds, and I found myself nearly overwhelmed by the urge to push. I again concentrated on the mechanics of transition and blew out forcefully and rapidly with each urge to push. Sometimes I'd feel like pushing for as long as thirty seconds, but I'd rehearsed the transition breathing well and it served me in good stead.

Around 10 A.M. the resident came back. I raised a hand in greeting, and somewhat taken aback by my happy mood, he saluted in return. I felt he was going to have good news for me and sure enough he told me I was fully dilated and could push now. What joy! What utter bliss! I was so happy not to have to hold back any more. My husband came back into the room to find me pushing and grinning from ear to ear. As we had been told, the expulsion contractions were quite bearable, coming every four to five minutes. Steve said my pushing did not have the precision it had in practice, but nevertheless it was quite effective if somewhat sloppy, because I could feel the baby moving down in the birth canal. In about thirty minutes the head had crowned and I was taken to delivery. I had my extra pillow with me and my doctor's permission to have my hands free. Steve and the doctor scrubbed up and joined me shortly.

From here on out things seemed to go very fast. Within two contractions, the head was born, followed rapidly by the arms. I felt the baby's body against my leg and in the next instant he was held in the air by the doctor and then placed on my abdomen. I was struck by how large he was and how nice and round his head was. He seemed beautiful to me. I was dumbfounded when I learned his weight. Ten pounds, fourteen and a half ounces. Twenty-three inches in length. My doctor said he was the biggest baby he had delivered without having to perform a caesarean section. And how beautifully the expulsion had gone. I thought I was having a seven-pounder.

By far the worst part of the whole experience was sitting up in bed in the recovery room feeling like a million dollars and listening to the anguished wails of three women who followed me into delivery. Later, I was the only woman brought a full lunch in the recovery room. I consumed it with relish.

Sincerely,
Peg K.

FROM THE HUSBAND

Dear Mrs. Bing:

I don't know if I have anything of importance to add to my wife's account, but I feel that birth à la Lamaze has given me a wonderful opportunity to participate in these events to an extent unthinkable otherwise, and could not let this opportunity pass to put my two cents in again at this stage.

It seems to me that we had several difficult obstacles to overcome in a successful application of the Lamaze technique. My wife's labor began fifteen days later than estimated, and repetition of the exercises was becoming extremely tedious. During the last week we missed several days of practice. The weather during most of my wife's pregnancy, especially July and August, was very hot and muggy and she was very uncomfortable. My wife's labor was almost entirely in her back and she experienced considerable trembling in transition. Finally, the baby, unbeknownst (fortunately) to us, was to weigh almost eleven pounds.

And yet, in spite of all this, the labor and delivery exceeded our best hopes in the way the techniques we learned served their purpose. Of course, only Peg can tell how the exercises effectively relaxed her and protected her from the intensity of the contractions. However, as I sat next to her in the labor room and tried to do the things I thought would help, I was more impressed than I ever had been with the difference a husband's presence can make. For example, such a simple thing as telling Peg what time it was: I always felt she responded with surprise—the time passed quickly, in view of her occupation with the exercises, and knowledge of the swift passage of time gave her added incentive to carry on. The visits of the doctor or resident seemed far apart and I am sure my presence, even without the timing of the contractions and occasional mopping of the brow, helped to break the desolation of four unsympathetic walls. Several times I found her flexing a leg or other limb and, apparently from excellent "conditioning," her responses to my reminders to let go were immediate.

My only regret was the rapid acceleration of events once Peg was fully dilated. I wanted to support and help her with the pushing, but shortly after she began to push I had to leave and get dressed for the delivery room. I joined her there about twenty minutes before the baby was born. She was in the best of humor and exchanging notable comments on the occasion with the resident. I was summoned to the front of the table to witness the crown of the baby's head. Our responses after that must have been very automatic, for neither of us have a very specific recollection of the events. The baby seemed to come very fast. Peg was not very impressed with the fact that it was a boy, apparently because subconsciously she had little doubt she was carrying a boy. I think the joy and emotional significance of these moments will not be so much what was felt during the birth itself as the wonderful memory and mental images we can invoke many times in the weeks (and I hope years) that follow.

Sincerely,
KARL K.

27

Laurie Elena

DEAR MRS. BING:

Despite the expected outcome, an emergency caesarean section, both Steve and I are glad to have had the psychoprophylactic training given us in your course. It turns out to be invaluable during labor, no matter what the final outcome. The whole idea of alleviating or banishing fear cannot be praised enough. Because once you've achieved the calm that training such as the Lamaze method brings, that calm is not easily shattered—not even by the ultimate of surprises, such as being wheeled into an operating room with only minutes' warning.

Also, all during labor, I could hear women in the rooms on either side of me who obviously had not had any kind of preparation for childbirth. They cried and screamed continuously, "Ay yi yi, I am dying, ay yi!" etc. This did not disturb my own equilibrium, much as it made me feel that the Lamaze or some similar method should almost be made obligatory for anyone who's going to bear children just so they won't feel they must suffer greatly.

It occurs to me that people who choose to attend classes or take any training similar to Lamaze method are perhaps the ones who least need such training. In our minds there is already the desire to learn as much as possible about childbirth and how to handle the fear or pain that is so often associated with it. This in itself may be the greatest step away from fear. Unfortunately, those women who are most fearful, most superstitious and who most need training are those least likely to receive it.

I'd certainly urge as widespread dissemination of the psychoprophylactic technique as possible.

When I expressed misgiving to my doctor for coming out from under the anaesthesia in a less than dignified manner (I seemed to have picked up the ay yi yi refrain from one of my labor roommates), he promptly countered by saying I'd come out amazingly well for having been thrown into what he called "the most terrifying situation" without any warning or preparation. Part of the credit, at least, must go to the calming influence of the Lamaze technique.

Recovery from the caesarean section has been fantastically rapid—up and walking within the shortest possible time, one day after.

The milk also came in one day later.

The baby is on a feeding-every-four-hours schedule.

And except for Wallace-LeMay, Nixon-Agnew, Humphrey-Muskie, *all's right with the world*. We're very happy with Laurie Elena, and apparently she with us—although she may not trust anybody over thirty days old.

Sincerely,

PATRICIA M.

EDITOR'S NOTE: Patricia was in labor for about thirteen hours. She only dilated 5 cm in spite of very strong contractions. The physician ruptured her membranes after several hours, after which labor stopped completely. Labor was then induced, and soon after, fetal distress occurred and Patricia was rushed into delivery for an emergency caesarean section. She certainly had no time to prepare herself mentally for this emergency, but as she describes above, she could manage even such an unforeseen event with calm and confidence in her physician. And, above all, she felt that even as far as she could use her training for a normal labor, she was highly successful and certainly never experienced any feelings of failure, depression or regret.

Tammy Adine

DEAR MRS. BING:

On Thursday afternoon, the day before my due date, the "bloody show" came and I very excitedly phoned the doctor, but since I didn't have any contractions he told me to sit tight and that it would be soon. I was so sure the baby would come on Friday, but she didn't, and that morning I woke up very depressed. It's a good thing that my husband is just nutty enough so that he always cheers me up. Friday was a normal day; that night we took our usual walk. At 4 A.M. I woke up and assumed that, as usual, I had to go to the bathroom, but before I got out of bed I could just feel and almost hear a kind of little pop and then I knew that the water bag had broken! It was dripping very slowly and I had no contractions for a while, so I sat in the bathroom with a good book and a clock for about ten minutes. When I started feeling a kind of pressure very low down every seven or eight minutes, I took my shower. I heard my husband get up, so I told him, and he got dressed and went to the kitchen to make some tea. It took me a while to dress because the pressure suddenly was coming every two or three minutes and I had to stop to breathe. I had to use second-phase breathing, and although the effleurage didn't help, just applying

31

strong pressure with my hands where I hurt did. All along we were very calm, assuming that we had plenty of time, since this was a first baby, but the doctor didn't agree and was upset that forty-five minutes had passed before I reached him by phone. He told us to leave immediately, so we left the tea, found a cab, and arrived at the hospital about 5 A.M.

Right from the start, the staff at the hospital was unbelievably helpful—not at all what I had anticipated. When the man in the admissions office asked if I wanted a wheelchair, I made a face, and he jokingly apologized for the "insult." We went upstairs before the forms were filled out; my husband went back down while I was being prepped. They already knew that I was using the Lamaze technique, and one nurse told the next, so I had no problem at all.

While I was being prepped I felt that I had to move my bowels, but nothing would come. The nurse told me to get back on the bed and she'd give me a small enema, but that didn't help either. The pressure was terribly strong, the breathing didn't help, and I was beginning to panic, especially since the doctor had examined me ten or fifteen minutes earlier and had said, "Five centimeters." So I thought that I still had five more cm to go. But I heard a woman screaming next door and I decided that if I wanted to see my baby born I'd just have to try once more. I started breathing again and this relaxed me. Then my mind started to function and I realized (or hoped) that I was probably feeling the baby's head. I called the nurse who took one look and said, "Oh my!" and ran to call the doctor. He came in grinning from ear to ear, saying, "I told you it would be a quick delivery, didn't I? And you probably would have stayed home longer!" In two seconds they had me in the delivery room. I never even got to unwrap a single lollipop! I forgot to take my pillows, but when I told the nurse she went back and brought them for me.

At this point one of the doctors found my husband, threw a green outfit at him and said, "Fast!" Elliot had not yet decided for sure whether or not he was going to come into the delivery room as well as the labor room, but he just didn't have any time to decide. There he was. Was I ever glad to see him, although he looked positively ridiculous in the green hairnet. He held my hand and he had to remind me to breathe, because all I wanted to do was push. Practicing, I had always found blowing very easy and the panting much more difficult, yet now, somehow, I couldn't make myself blow and I just panted like mad until *finally* I could push. I kept waiting for the cold shock of the solution to sterilize the vaginal area but the doctor used a spray which felt wonderful.

The baby's head came with the first push and the shoulders with the next. The afterbirth came by itself. We had entered the delivery room at 6 A.M.; our daughter was born at 6:15 A.M. I had closed my eyes while pushing, and when I opened them the doctor was just putting a beautiful, screaming, wet, pink, seven-pound baby on my stomach. I couldn't get over her perfectly round little head. She wasn't red or wrinkled or anything else I had expected. They gave her to me to hold while the doctor stitched the episiotomy, and no words could describe to you how I felt. The doctor had given me a local so I didn't feel the episiotomy at all, but I sure enough felt the stitches, and I let him know it. I don't remember all I said, but my husband informed me afterward that I was anything but friendly. Elliot and I just stared at the baby in elated disbelief—she was so beautiful, and it all happened so incredibly fast.

At 7 A.M. they moved me to the recovery room and my husband innocently followed. He was in there for half an hour before someone realized he didn't belong and asked him to leave. My toes were freezing, so he rubbed them for me. And being a good Lamaze husband, he also reminded me about the sphincter exercises. I could really feel my uterus as a hard ball that moved down.

In the delivery room I had been very thirsty but my lollipops were in the labor room and no one would give me a drink, so now I asked the doctor if I could have breakfast. At 8:45 A.M. they brought me a tray. The nurse proudly said, "That's what you get for having a prepared childbirth. Lamaze girls are always hungry." But I was really more thirsty than hungry. I almost felt guilty eating in there. The girl next to me was being given an intravenous. She had been awake for her delivery but not by choice, and she had many questions. She said that she knew that if she thought of something else the pain wouldn't be as bad, but she couldn't think of anything else to think about. Another woman in the recovery room was still asleep and the nurses were trying to arouse her.

Once in my room, I got out of bed, got cleaned up and started the sphincter exercises in earnest. Each day brought a great improvement, and by the third day only the change in position for sitting down or standing up was a bit uncomfortable. Every night the nurse offered me a sleeping pill, and I remember that it shocked me the first time because sleeping pills, in my mind, are for sick people and I felt marvelous.

Even though I had such a short labor, if it hadn't been for the classes I wouldn't have been able to relax and I wouldn't have known that it was the baby's head I felt. As a result of the classes, the birth of our daughter was an exciting and enjoyable *shared* experience that Elliot and I will never forget.

Sincerely,
MARLYNN D.

1519722

THE FATHER

DEAR MRS. BING:

I guess it's clear that I didn't have the baby, but I sure feel as if I did! From the nausea in the first three months to the delivery table and beyond, I found myself feeling a tremendous degree of empathy with Marlynn's moods and thoughts. But my reactions were often not hers, and what impressed me sometimes escaped her completely, so let me offer my version of the story.

The full consciousness of what was about to happen comes very slowly. Mentally, of course, I knew that my wife was pregnant and that eventually we would have a baby. I hoped that the baby would be healthy and the delivery easy. I also sometimes tried to imagine what being a father would be like. But somehow I *felt* very distant from the whole process—probably because my body was not physically involved.

Then Marlynn dragged me to some classes that her doctor insisted upon. At first I felt a little awkward and annoyed: after all, Marlynn was having the baby, so what did they need me for? And even though several of our friends who had gone through the Lamaze technique all talked about how important the husband's participation was, I frankly thought that they had been given a line and had swallowed it whole: What could a husband do to help his wife in such a situation when she was already going to be surrounded by people who were infinitely more competent in medicine than he? And furthermore, since I am queasy anyway, even if I were to go into the delivery room, I probably would faint and be more of a hindrance than a help. But I had already gotten used to humoring my wife during her pregnancy, so I consented to being dragged along.

Marlynn was ecstatic after the first few classes: I didn't become excited until the last few—but I *did* become excited, and that's what is remarkable. I still was not convinced that I was going to be any help; if anything, doing stupid things like timing Marlynn's make-believe contractions and shouting "Contraction begins" at her convinced me more than ever that my friends had deluded themselves, but good. But the truly miraculous nature of the birth process was mentally fascinating and, more important, knowing what was going on in Marlynn's body gave me some feeling of attachment to the whole thing. It was not a distant mystery any more. In fact, that feeling of attachment was probably the most important thing that the course did for me. And the tape of a labor and delivery and report of some other husband's experience generated an excitement that just had to catch on—and did. So, as we entered the last few weeks, I was going to go into the labor room, but I was still reserving judgment on that gory delivery room.

Now I have to mention something that I wasn't prepared for—in fact, the only thing that I wasn't prepared for. You hear all kinds of stories about how some babies come weeks early, others right around the due date, and others weeks late, but somehow you feel that whenever yours comes, it comes. But that's not what you feel when the second week of the ninth month rolls around—and that's certainly not what your wife feels. Marlynn, at any rate, began making plans about having the baby at various dates before her due date—half jesting, of course, but half serious too. It's a natural thing to do: you've been prepared for a very positive experience and have been waiting for nine months, and so you're keyed up and want it to come soon. Moreover, your friends and family add to the problems. They either ask you incessantly about how your wife is, or, if they have gone through this before, they try to be more considerate and don't call you at all—but get very excited whenever you call. I was really tempted to put a sign around my neck saying, "Not yet." They all mean well, of course, but it makes you more anxious. Then, when the real due date came and the baby was obviously not coming, Marlynn was terribly depressed. I had never seen her that way before. I tried to think of all kinds of trivial things that had nothing to do with the baby: I talked to her about our plans for the summer, I took her out with me to pick up the laundry, I took out one of our old camp songbooks and we sang and reminisced for a while, and—thank God—one of her college friends she hadn't seen for a while came over and they talked and talked and talked. Now remember that our baby was born only six hours after the due date; I shudder to think about how it would have been had it been later—as it might well have been. I don't know how one can prepare for this. I suppose it differs with every couple. But you should be prepared, and I mean especially the husbands.

Marlynn had the "bloody show" around noon on the day before her due date. Classes or no, I rushed home and was somewhat flustered. The doctor said to wait at least until contractions began, and they hadn't begun, so we took a walk, had supper, went to a movie and then for hot fudge sundaes (the first in months). But the water bag had not broken and Marlynn was still not feeling contractions, so we went to sleep. The next morning we woke up and still nothing else had happened, and that's when Marlynn began to be very depressed. The due date came and went. Late that night, however, I woke up to go to the bathroom and found Marlynn taking a shower. Her water bag had broken at 4 A.M. and she was having very mild contractions. She sat on the toilet while most of the water dripped off, reading Louis Nizer's *The Jury Returns* and doing the breathing for the first phase of labor. She asked me to make some tea, which I did, and meanwhile she called the doctor. I had to take the phone after Marlynn had said about two sentences to the doctor because she was having a contraction, and he was rather gruff. He asked me what we were doing home, and I frankly had no answer. At any rate, we left right away.

We found a taxi on Broadway almost immediately—quite amazing for 5 A.M. on a Saturday morning—and the driver was so tired that he didn't say anything about the funny breathing and rubbing Marlynn was doing in the back seat. I was thankful for his silence. When we got to the hospital the guard on duty had a broad smile on his face and escorted us to the admissions officer, who took us right upstairs and showed me where the waiting room was. He said that I would have to wait there until the baby was born, but when we exclaimed "Lamaze method of childbirth," he nodded and said, "Oh, yes, excuse me!" He then told me to kiss Marlynn "goodbye"—a rather gruesome way of putting it, I thought—and took me downstairs to sign some forms. We talked for about five minutes about nothing much, but he was really nice and put me at ease. As I was about to get on the elevator to go back upstairs, that nice guard asked me whether I wanted a nip, but I thanked him and refused. When I went into the waiting room, I saw a man there looking just like the expectant fathers you see in the movies. He looked terribly haggard, had smoked a lot, and was pacing back and forth. I really appreciated the course then because in comparison I was amazingly calm. I must have looked that way too, because when I introduced myself, he looked at me as if I was out of my mind. So I sat down and began reading Newsweek.

Five minutes later some man in a green uniform came in and asked for me. When I responded, he threw a similar green uniform at me and said, "Hurry!" I went into the room he indicated to change. The pants of the uniform were rather baggy, so I didn't know how they were supposed to go on. At first I took my slacks off and just put them on, but somehow that didn't look right, so I put mine back on and put the uniform over them. I still don't know whether that's right.

The doctor met me in the hall and gave me a hairnet and a nose mask and took me into the delivery room. I never saw the labor room because the baby was coming too fast. Now remember that I never really said that I was going to go into the delivery room. I suppose that by that time I was so excited I would have agreed anyway, but fortunately I never even had time to consider the alternative. I say "fortunately" because it really was the most thrilling experience of my life. I can finally understand why obstetricians are willing to get up so often at such monstrous hours.

When I got into the delivery room the doctor told me

39

to sit down on the stool next to Marlynn's shoulders. He had to tell me that twice, because I was a little surprised when I saw Marlynn. When I had left her, she had been quite calm, but by this time she was in the last stage of labor and working hard. The doctor told me to take her hand out of the strap and hold it. Just what I expected: The sum total of what I was to use from the course was holding my wife's hand! But I quickly discovered that that was not the case at all. Marlynn felt the urge to push several times when she was not supposed to and kept on asking the doctor if she could. Meanwhile she lost track of her breathing and was losing control. Primed by the courses to be a tyrant in the delivery room, I exclaimed, "Breathe!" as authoritatively but as softly as I could, and, by God, she did!

The doctor was delighted and told her that he should have arranged for more people to watch her. He then continued talking, describing everything that was happening. In the short time between contractions, Marlynn managed to tell me that I looked terrible in that green hairnet, and when the doctor said that I didn't look so bad, she told him that he didn't look so good either! I guess that indicates what kind of spirits she was in, even in the height of labor. Finally he told her to push, and boy, did she push! I saw the head come out, and on the second push the shoulders and the rest of the body came out. Tammy Adine came out pink and crying, seven pounds even. As soon as the baby was out, it was put on Marlynn's stomach and Marlynn began talking freely to the baby, to me, and to the doctor. I remember that when she asked him when the placenta was coming out, he said it already was out; she didn't even feel it. She complained about the stitches, but the doctor told her to stop insulting his golden hands.

40

When the stitches were finally sewn, Marlynn was wheeled to another room, which I later found out was the recovery room. I didn't know that at the time, however, so I just followed her in and talked with her for close to half an hour before a nurse asked me to leave. During that time Marlynn asked me when I wanted to have a second child—imagine, half an hour after she had just given birth to her first—and she had me rub her feet to get them warm. Her legs were still trembling a little, as they had been ever since we were in the cab, but it was slowing down considerably by now. She also remarked during that period, "Hey, I have a waistline!"

There remains but one thing that I should mention. The five days while Marlynn was in the hospital were exhilarating, frustrating and tiring. Exhilarating because I got to tell the story over and over again to very eager ears —and you can bet I did! Frustrating, because I got to see the baby only for about two minutes a day, and then she was behind the glass. And tiring, because I had to visit the hospital, go to my usual classes, and buy baby furniture in the same time in which I normally just go to school. As a result, those days were really quite annoying. But when the baby came home and things began to return to normal, it all became worth it. Of course, "normal" now will never quite be what normal used to be, but who would want it to be?

Sincerely,

ELLIOT D.

EDITOR'S NOTE: I always try to persuade the husband to let me know of his impressions after he supported his wife in labor. But it is not very easy to get a busy father to sit down and put his experiences and feelings on paper. I don't think the above report needs much of a comment from me—it shows so clearly what an important and shared experience can do to the warm and close relationship of husband and wife.

But I would like to insert here a note that one of the husbands wrote to me before his wife gave birth. It expresses what many young husbands feel. Here it is:

"It seems to me that a man and his wife deal with many difficult problems together during their marriage. It would be singularly unjust for a man to abrogate his responsibilities at this time, which is perhaps his wife's *most* difficult. Moreover, what kind of a paradox would it be, if he allowed his wife to enjoy alone the birth of their child? It may be the most beautiful, the most marvelous thing they have done. Why shouldn't he share in the enjoyment as well?"

Karen

●●●

DEAR MRS. BING:

The excitement began on the morning of the eighth when the doctor told me he was certain my labor would begin within twenty-four hours. By Friday morning, the ninth, however, nothing had happened and my husband went reluctantly to work, despairing of his long weekend off. I just sat down with a good book to pass the time until one in the afternoon, when with no warning at all I heard a loud bursting noise within me. There was a trickle of fluid and a sudden sharp contraction. The contraction had no sooner subsided when the phone rang—it was the doctor, wondering when I was ever going to get started at having this baby. I told him what had just occurred. He told me to time my contractions (they were four and three minutes apart), and by 2:30 I was at the hospital.

My contractions were strong and very close together from the beginning. I was never able to use the slow breathing at all and, as I remember it, used the very rapid panting and blowing almost the entire time (five hours) without becoming tired. I did ask for something to help relax me toward the end as I was very tense. But the small amount of Demerol I received in no way lessened my alertness or diminished the contractions. I was convinced, in fact, that

I had been given a placebo, but my husband assured me that I *was* more relaxed afterwards!

The one dark moment of the day came when I was in the midst of what I was sure was the transition phase: the contractions were of such strength that they literally lifted me off the bed; they were close to ninety seconds in length with a barely perceptible interval of rest. I was able, with great effort, to remain in control, but when an intern came in and told me I had reached only 6 cm of dilation, I announced to my husband that when my doctor returned I would ask him to put me to sleep as I couldn't imagine enduring anything stronger than those unbelievably powerful contractions. When the doctor examined me about ten minutes later, he agreed to do as I wanted but thought I might reconsider, since I was then at 9 cm and would be ready to deliver within a half hour.

I was so excited that I didn't bother to ask him how I had managed to go from 6 to 9 cm in ten minutes, but it turned out later that the young intern had been just a little off in his diagnosis of my progress.

Aside from this lapse, however, almost everyone at the hospital was unfailingly kind and helpful to me. The night of Karen's birth, in fact, was full of touching moments that only enhanced the ultimate beauty of the moment of her birth.

My husband, for example, was invited by the doctor to stand by his side during the delivery so he could really see what was happening, and before he left the delivery room the doctor congratulated us and told my husband that if we would arrange to have twins next time, he would let him deliver one of them!

Best of all, though, was the moment when, after a short wait in the delivery room, I was wheeled into my room to find awaiting me not just my empty bed and a long, sleepless evening, but, rather, my husband, resting in a chair, our newborn baby in his arms and, on a tray by my bed, a chicken dinner which the nurses had kept warm for me.

So there we were, less than an hour after our daughter's birth, alone together, alternately holding and admiring her and polishing off the food. Amid tears and sighs and incredible thoughts and looks, we began to make some calls, and thus it happened that my eighty-year-old grandmother, who I am sure thinks she has experienced everything, had the privilege that night of hearing her first great-grandchild, just forty-five minutes old, cry to her over the phone.

Needless to say, our experience with the Lamaze method of childbirth was, for us, most beautiful and rewarding, and we want to thank everybody who made it possible. I know that without the training I might never have succeeded as I feel I did, and certainly I would not be looking forward as I now am, to not just "having" but to actively giving birth, hopefully, to two or three more babies as lively and beautiful as our little Karen.

Sincerely,
Lynne M.

Laura

- -

DEAR MRS. BING:

You asked for a blow-by-blow of every one of our labors, so I suppose by now you are very bored with accounts of how well the breathing worked. So here follows a letter of respite from such comments.

I have a terrible confession to make: I did hardly any breathing whatsoever. The reason for this heinous disregard for all I was taught had nothing to do with panic or the like. You always stressed the importance of not starting to pant madly until you needed control. This never happened, and so I literally breezed through the delivery sans anesthetic and actually enjoyed (practically) every minute of it.

Around noon of the sixth of November I started to notice the strangest tightenings in my lower abdomen. I concluded that they were some sort of gas pains because it was a full two weeks until my due date. But, conditioned as I had been to watch the clock, I was alarmed to find that they were ten minutes apart (every once in a while fifteen or twenty). I did all I could to convince myself that this wasn't really "it," but when at 3 P.M. I discovered that I was staining, I did the distance from the bathroom to the phone in Olympic record time. The doctor told me to go on with my normal activities, eat a normal supper, and to call him back when the contractions came five minutes apart.

So I took a shower, and by then (about 5 P.M.) I couldn't bend down very well to dry my legs. This should have given me a clue that I wasn't just effacing any more, but my thought patterns were far from logical. The contractions already were five minutes apart at 6 P.M., and 6:30 found me gingerly mincing around the house, packing my totally unprepared hospital gear into the smallest suitcase in creation. The doctor thought it would be a good idea to go to the hospital early so that when I registered I wouldn't be in any great discomfort. So off I went in a jolly enough mood until in the car I clocked in a contraction only two and a half minutes from the last. I still didn't need that fabled control, so I just relaxed my whole body every time a contraction came and sort of figured I was letting nature take its course.

At the hospital I was offered a wheelchair, which I really didn't need, since it was by now more uncomfortable for me to sit than to stand and walk. So I walked into the labor room and was left to get undressed and leave a urine sample (that was easier said than done!) and various other things. I told no one my contractions were less than three minutes apart because no one asked.

So there I was, approaching my point of no control (at last) and cranking up the bed myself, and never taking my eyes off that clock. An intern sauntered in, very relaxed, and said he would give me a routine examination. He didn't believe the two-minutes-apart part until he examined me and the look of relaxed unconcern was wiped off his face in a split second. It even disconcerted me. He said, "Oh, you're doing marvelously!" I asked how many fingers. He said three. I asked something about "Hasn't the doctor been called yet?" Then ensued a heated discussion on fingers and centimeters and how many of each

47

you need for full dilation. Finally (I thought) we had cleared up the subject and learned I was only three centimeters dilated. As it turned out, though, it *had* been three fingers, but he didn't want to scare me, since my doctor was still at home, unalerted, watching the football game. He told us later that when they finally got through to him I was 8 cm dilated; he put on his pants backward and tore over to the hospital, ready to congratulate the interns on how well they had done without him. About half an hour before I went to the delivery room, the good doctor sprinted in, examined me, and said, "You are fully dilated, you can start pushing." This had been labor? And it was all over? And no breathing? It seemed too ridiculous. I told him he was out of his mind, which started him laughing. Convinced he was a maniac, I started pushing.

And so, labor more or less over, I guess most people would say, "And the rest was easy." The only difference with me was that my labor was so easy that the pushing part seemed practically impossible—sort of an "irresistible force against immovable object" type of feeling. I never thought it would work. But it took relatively few pushes to get the job done, so I guess there again I was lucky. I found that even though I hadn't had much of a chance to practice it, I knew instinctively which muscles to use and what to do to make each contraction most effective. It took only about six or seven contractions for the head. When that was out, I was under the impression that the whole baby had been born, it was such a relief. The doctor said something about a beautiful baby, so I immediately asked what it was. He told me, "It looks to me like a boy," which made me feel awfully good (as the opposite answer would have done). About ten seconds later, however, he told me, "One more push for the shoulders," which was kind of a letdown. I lifted myself up again (I

48

got terribly stiff arms from the pushing) and so became the only mother in history who, without having twins, had a boy and a girl at one delivery. After the head, everything really went very smoothly and I had a very blue baby girl who turned pink the minute she let out a very apathetic little moan. (I thought that was the most appropriate greeting 1968 deserved anyway.) Then they were all over me, one nurse putting ink on my finger for the paper with the baby's footprints on it, another at my other arm smearing on alcohol in preparation for a belated shot of Demerol, and the doctor pushing down on my stomach, asking if I had one more push left. I had plenty left—I had been spared the hours some people spend in the delivery room, pushing ineffectually (maybe just incorrectly?).

I could write you pages about the baby and about all the postpartum rigmarole, but that isn't what you probably want. I think I know now why girls in our society are so indoctrinated about the agonies of childbirth. People who have "been through it" simply relish recounting every gory detail. I found this rotten trait even more irritating since I acquired it myself. Not that I embellish my success story (I consider it that) with all sorts of gruesome accounts of how bloody awful it was. In fact, I was entirely too busy at the end and entirely too fascinated with everything that was going on around me to notice any great discomfort. Mrs. Bing, it was really great. I'm looking forward to the second. I hope you enjoyed this little missive as much as I enjoyed typing it with so many many errors.

I'll be back someday for a refresher, and meanwhile, thanks for everything.

Sincerely,
JENNIFER F.

49

Deena Beth

•••

DEAR MRS. BING:

It had finally come: August 10, the date I expected my baby to arrive, and—no baby. With each successive day of waiting I became more and more depressed; however, we continued exercising and breathing. I had become proficient at the breathing techniques and was eager to apply all our knowledge to help our baby enter the world.

Sixteen days after my due date, my long-awaited labor began at 9 P.M. I could not believe that it was happening and had to be assured by my husband that it was the real thing. I quickly packed my last-minute things and attempted to go to bed. However, I seemed to have back labor and I was so uncomfortable that I could not sleep.

The contractions were coming about twenty minutes apart and we knew we had a long way to go. We took pencil and paper and proceeded to keep an accurate account of each contraction. The hours started to pass and we saw no pattern emerge. The contractions went from twenty minutes apart to five minutes to fifteen to seven. It was sporadic all through the night but became a little more intense at about 1:30 A.M., so I started my chest breathing. At this point I insisted that my husband get some sleep and he eagerly complied with my request. By

7 A.M. I was still in preliminary labor and the contractions were extremely sporadic. I called the doctor and he told us to go directly to the hospital. (Later I learned that the doctor thought that I was in transition labor at that point because so many hours of contractions had elapsed.) We grabbed my suitcase, lollipops, washcloth, tennis-ball can (for my back labor) and a camera to catch all those exciting facial expressions while breathing.

At about 7:30 A.M. we arrived at the hospital. I was sent directly to the labor room and was to be prepped. I refused to be prepped until I had been examined by my doctor. (I knew that I had a long way to go and did not want to spend all that time in the hospital. If I were prepped they would not allow me to leave, therefore I asked to be examined first.) I was told by the head nurse that he was in the delivery room and would not be out for a while. My second request was to have my husband sent up to me to the labor room and this was also refused.

After a half hour of waiting in the "howling ward," I decided to take radical measures. If the hospital would not cooperate, then I was taking things into my own hands. I proceeded to dress and attempted to leave the labor area to go down to my husband when the head nurse came running after me. I told her that I was leaving because my husband was not sent up to my room. Half frightened and half angry, she insisted that she knew what was best for me and demanded that I return to my room and undress. I replied, "Only I know what is best for me." I then saw my doctor emerge from the delivery room, mask and all. He started to yell, saying, "What are you carrying on about?" and took me to an examining room. He could not understand why I came to the hospital when his orders were not to call him until contractions were three

51

minutes apart. He had obviously forgotten that he had told me to come to the hospital at 7 A.M. and that I had had sporadic contractions all night long. I told him what had taken place and the length of my labor. At that point he broke my water. Now I had to stay.

I was prepped and given pitocin intravenously to stimulate the contractions. My husband was finally sent up. After I had told him of my experience, he related his frantic actions while waiting for the nurse to advise him that it was time to join me in the labor room. He had already made a pest of himself by demanding that he be issued a pass and taken to the labor room. Both the medical secretary and elevator operator were at him for his "pushy" and unorthodox behavior.

Contractions started coming at regular five-minute intervals and I was told I was dilated 3 cm. By twelve o'clock I would probably have my baby. The most uncomfortable part, however, was the back labor, which the tennis-ball can helped to alleviate somewhat. My position throughout the entire twenty-four hours remained the same: leaning slightly forward while in a sitting position.

Before I continue my experiences I must interject some important points about the hospital staff and their attitude toward patients. Prior to our arrival we were told that the hospital would be very cooperative; however, our fourteen hours spent there proved otherwise. It was extremely crowded this particular day, with several women put into the same room, and I was refused a private labor room. Each time a woman was brought into my room, my husband was asked to leave. It is a good thing that we were Lamaze-oriented. My husband knew how important it was for us to be together and he antagonized practically the whole staff by insisting that we be given a private room. He was not only forced to leave my room but was told to wait downstairs in the waiting room until a room was available. On several occasions he "acquired" a pass and returned to the labor area to insist that a private room be made available immediately. The elevator operator threatened to call the security guard to have my husband removed bodily.

Finally, after many heated arguments regarding how important it was for my husband to be with me in order that we be able to utilize the Lamaze technique, a private room was provided.

The nurses were awed by our performance, as they had little knowledge or experience with the Lamaze method. All three women, who had been wheeled into the room I occupied before, were heavily sedated, yet they continued to cry, as I quietly went about my business of breathing and massaging each time I had a contraction.

At about 2 P.M. I was examined by a resident: still only 3 cm dilated. Both my husband and I knew that something was wrong. The doctor told us that the baby's heartbeat was a little rapid and that he was concerned. He stated that he would have a resident periodically check the baby's heartbeat as he had to return to his office. He said that I was doing just fine—performing like a champ. He left for his office, to return again at 7 P.M.

By 7 P.M., after two hours of receiving oxitocin to make the contractions more effective, they were now coming every minute and lasting ninety seconds. Dilation: between 3 and 4 cm. The resident examined me less frequently, thus reinforcing my frustration and fear.

How depressing all this was. I truly believed that I was never going to have a baby. I was ready to give up the breathing, the effleurage, the tennis-ball can and submit

53

to anesthesia. I so badly wanted to get some rest and forget all this.

But something prompted me to continue: it was the love, warmth, respect and admiration in my husband's eyes. These many hours spent together like this were creating a stronger bond between us. We needed each other very badly at this moment and I would not leave my husband by submitting to medication.

When the doctor returned at 7 P.M., he stated what we already feared. A caesarean section would be performed around 9 P.M. if there was no progress. At 9 P.M., when a final decision for a section was made, my husband reluctantly left me and remained alone in the waiting room. For him this was probably the most difficult part of the whole experience—not knowing what was happening to me.

At 9:38 P.M. Deena Beth was born by caesarean section.

You might wonder of what use the Lamaze method was to me and why I am so grateful for having experienced part of it—knowledge and labor without fear. Unfortunately the hospital staff could not have been more uncooperative. We received no help, no comfort, and little understanding. We were told very little about my condition and what was actually taking place.

Only because my husband and I were so knowledgeable and knew precisely what to expect throughout labor were we able to realize that there were complications. We were able to ask questions and insist upon answers from our doctor and the staff. Labor thus became a shared experience, and I can only imagine what the birth of our beautiful little girl would have been. You see, she was brought to me the following day, and as happy and as pleased as I was with her, I still felt that I missed something—bringing her into the world myself with the help of my husband. I know that we would have done a superb job.

It might not be necessary for me to have a section next time. It is a lot easier perhaps not to have to go through with labor, but we feel strongly that we want to be together when we give birth to our child, and we will certainly try it the second time around.

Sincerely,
CONNIE C.

Elizabeth

●━━━━━━━━━━━━━━━━━━━━━━━━━━━━━━━━━━●

DEAR MRS. BING:

I must first confess that I came to Lamaze as a cynic, convinced that this was but one more plot of the feminists to emasculate the male by dragging him down into their own private suffering. Quite influenced by Spencer Tracy and Gary Cooper, I was eager instead to chain-smoke all night, pace the floor with other men of good cheer, gaze out the quaint little window at the moon, speak to the universe, and think how I would make this world a better place for my child to live in.

It was along about the third lesson that a basic instinct began to tug at my necktie—that of almost all primitive men—to be a part of their mates' experience during labor. Having just researched several African tribes, I found it almost universal that men in some way participate—albeit vicariously—in the actual birth process. At any rate, I began to get excited about being around for the big event —but still was not convinced, mind you, that I'd have actually anything to do. Surprise. Was I wrong!

Alice's labor began as "gas pains" in the middle of the night, and we were hospital bound at around 4 A.M. I advise that all husbands arrange their wives' labor to begin in the dim hours. The sight of a small, motionless Buddha in the passenger seat, gracefully effleuraging and breathing, her face illuminated only by the lights of the dashboard, is an image forever etched in my memory. Really quite surrealistic, and quite beautiful.

At the hospital, contractions were light, dilation progressing. I went to the commissary with our doctor and had breakfast in the company of five interns. I don't advise eggs for breakfast for the husbands in labor. Hard to look at. The interns didn't help much. They talked about "innards." I covered my eggs with a napkin, and headed back upstairs.

Hard contractions had developed—and Alice was in back labor. We hadn't been diligent about our back labor practice, and I was at first squeamish about laying hands on a woman in labor. But it was no problem. The height of the bed made it immeasurably easier than I had imagined it while practicing on the floor. I sat on the edge, and supported Alice's back, while she assumed the side-saddle knee-chest position. The proverbial urge to push came early, intensely, and was to be the cornerstone of the seven hours of labor that followed.

I became a one-man band, actually breathing and blowing louder than Alice, my right hand pounding out the rhythm on her arm, while my left hand did a wild effleurage on her back. Her urge was almost unbearable, and occasionally she gave way, but I put her back on the track by saying firmly, "Go back! Start over! Stay on top!"— and other such inspired remarks. Twice I had to redirect her attention to the flower on the window sill by pointing at it; but once it was refixed, she stayed with it.

Transition came without knocking first. And we slipped into the breathing quite naturally. Alice, incidentally, was never so good at breathing as she was during actual labor.

Many times during practice she had become discouraged, but somehow, with real contractions, it was easier. She was panting like a Saint Bernard running for a bowl of Friskies.

The most exciting moment came for me at the end of transition, when, with my hand against Alice's back, I felt the baby turn—shoulders, elbows and all. How fantastic to know what it was!

I was not permitted into the delivery room, but it only took twenty minutes, and Alice claimed it was sheer heaven. She described defying the urge to push like trying to hold in a huge enema—and when she was allowed to let go—well, it's a feeling that all of us who have had enemas fondly remember.

The baby was, I thought, quite beautiful, and I was overwhelmed at the sight of it—so much more so because I felt *I* had done it. I honestly feel as though I was one-half responsible for it—and how great it was to have been able to share something so important with Alice. If that sounds soppy, don't forget I was a cynic—and like a re-formed alcoholic, I can't stop preaching the gospel.

Vital statistics: Seven-pound, nineteen-inch baby girl, born of a 105-pound, five-foot mother.

Got some flack from the delivery-room nurses, but at the time couldn't have cared less.

Thanking Pavlov—and his disciples, Lamaze and all Lamaze teachers—I remain profoundly grateful.

Sincerely,
DAVID S.

Nicholas

DEAR MRS. BING:

I am sorry it took so long to get this report to you, but I'm sure you'll understand when I say that things have been hectic around here.

Nicholas is gorgeous, but what a time-consumer!

It became routine, in those final weeks of my pregnancy, to make several predawn trips to the bathroom. So I wasn't surprised, when, at 4:30 A.M. on October 31st, I groped my way in the darkness (my husband was sleeping soundly) to the john. What *did* surprise me, once there, was the realization of a menstrual-like cramp. I had heard that early labor sometimes starts out this way; I was not sleepy any more. . . .

In another ten minutes a second cramp came along. Wait, I told myself, before you get excited. After all, the baby wasn't due yet for another two weeks, and weren't first babies always late? Besides, there were no other signs; my water hadn't broken, there was no bloody show, no mucus plug. When a third cramp came again about ten minutes later, I decided to run a bath. That would calm down what was most likely a case of wishful thinking.

The running water roused my husband. "Mmmmphh?" he said, which I interpreted to mean, "What's up?"

"Nothing," I told him, deliberately keeping my voice calm. "It's just that I think I'm having contractions, but it's probably only a false alarm. Go back to sleep."

To my annoyance he did precisely that!

The twinges (they weren't strong enough to be "pains") kept coming all the while I was soaking in the comfortably warm water. And suddenly, up bobbed a small thick clot of mucus. The mucus plug? I wasn't sure; there wasn't a tinge of blood. But I decided to be on the safe side and got out of the tub in a hurry.

Something was definitely happening, and a zillion thoughts flooded my mind: My hair needed washing, my suitcase needed packing, the laundry needed ironing. . . . This *couldn't* be real labor!

But the cramps continued . . . now ten minutes apart, now eight, now ten again, now seven. . . .

At 5:15 A.M. I washed and set my hair. I packed my suitcase just as the first gray streaks of daylight came filtering through the darkness. My Lamaze bag, which I had thought to assemble a week before, was double-checked: lollipops, washcloth, chapstick, talcum powder. Everything seemed A-Okay. Then, as an afterthought, I put your book, *Six Practical Lessons for an Easier Childbirth*, on top of the suitcase. (It stayed with me, a sort of security blanket in hard cover, all throughout labor!)

At 7 A.M. I crept back into bed and began to time the contractions, all the while grinning to myself, basking in the glow of "This is it!"

But was it? I still wasn't sure. Even though they were now coming every five minutes, the contractions were so mild I hadn't even needed to begin my deep breathing exercises.

Half an hour later my husband woke, refreshed from

a sound night's sleep. (That made *one* of us, anyway, refreshed!)

"The contractions are coming every five minutes," I announced joyously.

It was his turn to snap to. "Call the doctor!" he ordered.

"But they are so mild," I protested, "I don't know if I should."

Allan insisted. So, more to allay his fears than mine, I dialed the doctor's number. It was 7:55 A.M.

"Remember that chat we were supposed to have on my next visit?" I said to the doctor. (He was to have instructed me, at that time, just when to call him, what signs to look for, etc.) "Well," I said, "I think we'd better have it now."

He asked when the contractions had started, how frequently they were coming, and the duration of each. Then he told me to call back in an hour.

By 8:30 A.M. they were coming at four-minute intervals and lasting about thirty-five to forty seconds. They had become a teeny bit stronger. I decided to begin my deep breathing exercises.

"Better come to the hospital," the doctor said when I called him back.

"Do you really think it's necessary?" I wanted to know, still not convinced that this was the real thing. And I'd hate to be sent home again with false labor!

"Well," the doctor pointed out, "things seem to be speeding up rather than slowing down. I think we'd better check to make certain."

But in the taxi, sure enough, the contractions abated. "Oh, great," I complained, feeling like a fool.

"At least we'll have gotten a little ride out of it," my husband said—the eternal optimist.

The labor room turned out to have a lovely view of Central Park. It was a beautiful autumn morning, all amber and orange and Halloweeny . . . Halloween. Was this to be a trick-or-treat baby?

The doctor came in as soon as I had gotten undressed and into one of those unpretty hospital gowns. "You're four cm dilated," he said, smiling, after examining me.

"You're kidding!" I exclaimed, amazed and delighted at once. So it was not my imagination after all.

"The nurse will be in to prep you, and then your husband will be allowed upstairs. I'll be back in an hour or so, to see how things are going."

"Fine," I said. And it was fine. I felt marvelous! Here I was in the labor room, in the second phase of the first stage of labor, my Lamaze bag ready on the table beside me, and Mrs. Bing's book under my arm.

A student nurse—she couldn't have been older than nineteen—strode briskly into the room. (Why do all student nurses walk as if they have springs in their shoes?)

"Good morning," she said, eying me warily. (I could hear her thinking, What will this one be like? Will she give us much trouble?) "I'm your nurse, Miss B., and I'll be with you throughout your labor."

That was a surprise! I had no idea I was to be assigned my very own nurse for the whole thing. I wasn't too happy about it either. All these months I had imagined just my husband and myself, in a cozy little ménage à deux, with occasional visits from the doctor. . . . Well, I sighed, she's here to learn, so be nice for the benefit of educated youth. I reached for my Lamaze bag and offered her a lollipop.

When the prep was over, my husband was notified, and in he walked in his sterile white gown. He looked so handsome in it, I told him he had missed his calling;

instead of an architect, he should have been a doctor.

I introduced him to "our" nurse, and we all settled down to what would eventually be an afternoon of waiting.

There was a big clock on the wall facing my bed, which was nice, insofar as I could literally see time slipping by; but as the day wore on, and the contractions grew in intensity, it was my husband's face I sought as he called out, "Fifteen seconds, thirty, forty-five . . ." And when I took a cleansing breath at the end of each contraction, he did too.

True to his word, the doctor appeared about 11:30 A.M. to announce that I was 6 cm dilated. I was ecstatic: more than halfway through the first stage, and I was still deep breathing!

"Shouldn't I begin to pant?" I asked the doctor warily. Maybe there was something wrong—it seemed too easy.

"Begin only when you feel you need to," he answered, adding, "It varies from woman to woman. Some begin panting when they are two cm dilated; others not until seven."

I needn't have worried about not needing to pant. About half an hour later I suddenly found that deep breathing was not enough; that I was tensing up, forgetting to relax. Yet I was reluctant to admit that panting was what was necessary now; there is something very attractive about being a Trojan and all that. . . .

The nurse had gone to lunch (apologetically) and so had my husband. It was the first time I had been left to myself since I had come to the hospital, and, frankly, it was quite pleasant. I'm sure the nurse meant well, but every time I looked she was doing something for me: taking my blood pressure or listening to the fetal heart beat,

63

or checking to see if my water had broken (it had not) or looking for some "show," etc.

Go ahead, I persuaded myself, pant. I did. It worked. Once more I felt able to relax, to lean back and enjoy myself. It sounds crazy, I know, but it *was* enjoyment. Putting into practice things you had been trained for and seeing positive results—there is nothing like it!

One thing I craved and couldn't have was water. Lollipops are fine, but they are not exactly thirst-quenchers. I kept envisioning tall glasses of cold lemonade.

During the afternoon, other nurses kept popping in. Word had evidently gotten around that there was someone having a "natural childbirth" in this room, and they wanted to see for themselves how well I was bearing up. (The bearing *down* part came later!) I began to feel a bit like Exhibit A in a courtroom.

That was another surprise, as a matter of fact. It seems that natural childbirth is still something of a rarity today (most of my friends have had it, and that is the reason I assumed it was so widespread), with the majority of women coming down from the delivery room completely zonked out.

At 3 p.m. the doctor came in again and, after another examination, decided it was time to break the membranes. "That will speed things up," he said. I was glad to hear that, because I was getting tired. Laughing and joking with my husband and the nurses was great for my morale, but I had forgotten one of the basic tenets of prepared childbirth: conserve your energy between contractions!

The breaking of the membranes was painless enough, but the doctor wasn't kidding when he said it would speed things up. Now the contractions came every two minutes, then every one and a half minutes. And I don't care what natural childbirth advocates say, they were *painful!* Bearable but, as the hour wore on, less and less so.

The next time the doctor examined me he said I was about 9 cm dilated—well into transition. It couldn't get much worse. I knew that. But knowing it didn't make it easier.

I began to feel panicky. I began the pant-blow technique, even though I hadn't the slightest urge to push. That helped some, but now I really was tired and perspiring and thirsty and I knew that a few more hours of this —even one hour—I could not stand. It seemed that there was no let-up at all between contractions. The young nurse, her hand on my stomach, kept saying, "The contraction is finishing now." And I, irritated at her telling me, retorted, "It is not! It's still there!"

The heck with natural childbirth! I'd had it, and now I wasn't liking it one bit. "Tell the doctor to give me something," I demanded.

The doctor came in, this time in cap and gown. "Are you sure you want something?" he asked.

"I'm sure, I'm sure!" I said frantically. It was close to 4 P.M. None of us knew—not even the doctor—that the baby would be born in eighteen minutes.

I was given a shot of Demerol, which did absolutely no good whatever. It was much too late.

"Do you feel any urge to push?" the doctor asked.

"No," I said.

"Try anyway."

I did. It hurt.

He examined me again. "No, there is still a tiny rim of cervix left," he said.

But then suddenly, a minute or so later, the urge was there! Very slight, at first, then, with a succeeding contraction, more and more undeniable. "I have to push!" I cried triumphantly. Then, "But I have forgotten how!"

The doctor reminded me; the nurse reminded me; and my husband reminded me—all at once!

I pushed, took a breath and pushed again. One, two, three more times.

"Well," said the doctor, "it's all over but the shouting —the baby's shouting!"

Then my husband was motioned to the foot of the bed. "I can see the baby's head!" he said, his face aglow with wonder.

All traces of panic disappeared promptly when the doctor said, "Okay, we'll take you into delivery now."

Unfortunately that was as far as it went for my husband. At this hospital the attitude is still a conservative *no* to husbands in the delivery room—and how unfair!

Once on the delivery table, with my legs in stirrups (much more comfortable than pushing in the labor-room bed!) the doctor began to arrange a mirror on the opposite wall so that I could watch the birth of my baby.

"A little to the right," I directed. "No, now a little to the left . . . that's fine!"

And then I could see for myself the baby's head, dark and wet, coming closer and closer into the world. . . .

After the next three or four pushes the doctor performed the episiotomy and the baby's head was born, almost that very second. I heard a soft whimper, then a little cry. Not even fully born yet, and crying already! It was 4:18 P.M. exactly—almost twelve hours from the onset of labor.

"Don't push for just a minute," the doctor instructed, as he was about to deliver the shoulders. I panted and blew, panted and blew, until the final order to push came.

"You'll have to tell me the sex of the baby," the doctor said, holding up a squirming little body.

"It's a boy!" I shouted gleefully. It was the only time I had shouted that day.

He was beautiful. Long lashes and dark hair and artist's hands. I couldn't take my eyes away from him for a second. I resented the intrusion when the doctor held up the placenta, seconds later, for me to look at.

I did not feel a thing all the while the doctor was stitching the episiotomy.

I felt nothing except intense pride and a profound sense of accomplishment equal to nothing I felt in my life before.

Sincerely,
SUSAN T.

Lisa

DEAR MRS. BING:

I have thought of you, mentally written you, and thanked you so many times, but only now I am finally putting my thoughts into a letter.

In August 1961, while a student at a New York school of nursing, I wrote my obstetric case study on a woman who used the then very unique Lamaze method. I was so impressed with her—not only her seeming physical ease but also her attitude of complete involvement in her child's birth—that I decided that when my time came, the Lamaze method was for me. I sent my term paper to you and was again inspired, this time by your enthusiasm.

Finally my chance was to come. Last year my husband (then a first-year resident in internal medicine) and I were living in Seattle, Washington, and I received my obstetrical care through the University Hospital out-patient clinic. My doctor's attitude was, "Let's just see what happens in delivery." I felt he was flexible enough to go along with what I wanted.

I was working and did so until the week before I delivered, and—well, I just never did decide to attend the classes.

I had two sources for self-instruction. The first was the Seattle Public Library, where, to my amazement, they had the books specifically filed in the librarian's office! The second was another physician's wife, who had graduated three years ahead of me at Cornell. She too was self-taught, and she had had her second child in India. After walking to the delivery room she found there were no stirrups or leg supports at all on the delivery table; luckily she had practiced her pushing and was able to proceed without difficulties. She was an excellent source of enthusiastic teaching.

Again, however, I procrastinated; I was convinced the baby would be late, and it was always "tomorrow night" that I would begin a regular routine of practicing. I did practice sporadically, and after thinking about the Lamaze method all those years, I felt prepared.

Finally the big moment! After a day hiking with my husband and father-in-law, I fell into bed refreshingly exhausted. Ten minutes later I rose in disbelief—it was a day before my due date and I just couldn't or wouldn't believe that this was it. About two hours later—about 2 A.M.—I woke my husband. Contractions were about every ten minutes and, I felt, quite strong. I had previously grabbed my Xeroxed copy of the instructions from my book and had been doing the deep-breathing exercise, more for practice, as I really didn't need any control breathing yet.

Between 3 and 5 A.M. seemed to be the most difficult period for me. I switched to the faster breathing because I became more uncomfortable, but really, I think, because it gave me more to do. The doctor later said that this may have been when I was doing the real stretching of my cervix, and I therefore had more discomfort. Personally I think it was because the whole world was asleep and there I was . . . tired and awake.

At this point I think I should mention my dear wonderful husband. It seems every doctor has something that makes him uncomfortable. Well, after Terry had fainted at three deliveries as a student, he was finally able to watch and then quite competently deliver many babies. Now it was two years since he had delivered those babies, and he said he just wouldn't feel comfortable coming into the delivery room. I wonder how much of his previous attitude was caused by having to attend as a student the labors and deliveries of untrained, uncontrolled and screaming women. Anyway, I didn't think it was fair to push him as he was sensitive about it already. He was a wonderful help during labor just by his presence.

At about 5 A.M. the sun rose gloriously over Lake Washington, and my spirits soared. By 7 A.M. I was 7 cm dilated. I was then seen by my doctor, who then ordered pelvimetry X rays. He also offered me some Demerol which I refused because, honestly, it didn't hurt that much. Maybe it was because in between contractions I was able to relax so completely. During the X rays I asked the technician at one point if he'd "please wait until the contraction is over" before he put me into another weird position. He seemed shocked to learn that I was in labor. I'm not complimenting myself, only showing what a wonderful control the Lamaze technique provided.

Back on the delivery floor, my doctor told me that the baby was still very high and that he hoped that I could push the baby down, also that "she" was in a breech position. (The advantages of a breech; I knew already I was going to have a little girl!) There was a possibility of a caesarean section if I could not push the baby low enough. I had such confidence in my doctor and was so excited about being in labor that I was not really scared by the possibility of a section, only disappointed that I might not be able to see my baby born. At this point my doctor also asked me how I had been able to keep such a good control during my labor. Hurray! I pulled out my Xeroxed copy and briefly, between contractions, preached the Lamaze technique.

At 9:30 A.M. I was 9 cm dilated. I was beginning to feel a little tired and uncomfortable and therefore accepted 25 mg of Demerol, which was given intravenously.

I was then taken to the delivery room. The possibility of a section was still present, so I was as cooperative as I could be.

I pushed for an hour—the most physically taxing work I had ever done in my life. Here I needed help; the contractions seemed to be one on top of the other. Fortunately the delivery nurse was excellent and was able to channel my efforts into effective pushing. I asked the doctor if ten more pushes would do it—it seemed necessary at this time to have a goal. He said ten would be fine, and three contractions later my daughter—bruised bottom, but beautiful—was delivered. I am sure you hear over and over how exhilarating an experience it is, thanks to Dr. Lamaze!

And then the overwhelming closeness when my husband came in after first seeing the baby!

I wonder about next time . . . and already there is a definite next time. And next time I would like my husband to share the experience with me, and I think I will then have so much confidence in my own performance that I can reassure my husband and also make him feel confident and calm, and happy to share the experience with me.

Sincerely,
JOAN F.

A Husband's Account

EDITOR'S NOTE: I was asked to speak at a symposium at a State University school of nursing. The professor who had invited me to speak had also invited a young couple who had successfully used the Lamaze technique for their two children to report on their experiences. The husband gave his account, and I was listening, enthralled, to what he had to say. I asked him later if he could write down his thoughts for me because at that time I was already collecting material for this book. He promised, and finally his account came, and I will reproduce it here in full, because he expressed his thoughts and feelings in such lucid terms that I felt I wanted to share his letter with you.

DEAR MRS. BING:

When attempting to understand the support needed by the mother it seems necessary that the hospital staff directly involved realize the purpose of the parents in electing the Lamaze method. Obviously they have not done so for comfort's sake. No one in a reasonable frame of mind would choose such a method if freedom from pain were the only concern, since chemical means are so much more efficient in this respect. Indeed, chemical analgesia and anesthesia can be so complete as to deny any consciousness of the event at all, and herein lies the reason for rejecting them. We do not care to sleep away our lives, nor sacrifice particularly important moments, nor yet modify the quality of these moments so much that their value to us is likewise modified.

Let us remember that in most pre-Renaissance or traditional cultures, what was thought of as the "good life" was not understood in terms of material ease. Those experiences that we can only call "spiritual" gave the desired mode of life its value, and these were such as love, friendship, wisdom, morality, justice, temperance and something we think of today as "naturalness"—a close relation to nature. The birth of a child was a privilege as well as a labor, and the experience of giving birth was not easily rejected. Through it both father and mother participated in the process of the cosmos; through it particularly, for our very term "nature" is derived from *natus*, birth. To give up such an experience because it can only be obtained through physical discomfort is like refusing the winter because it is cold or the summer because it is hot.

In our technologically-minded society it is easy to overlook spiritual values and misunderstand the purposes of those who still share them. We like to "get things done" and often overlook that one may appreciate the process as well as its result. Those who have chosen the Lamaze method have done so for spiritual reasons; they desire an experience and hope to preserve the proper quality of that experience. Thus it does not help either mother or father to feel that these values are not shared by the doctor or the nurse. If the staff is felt to be "going along because they have been paid to do so," there can hardly be any feeling of human community in the labor or delivery room. The mother needs more than sympathy with her physical situation—she requires sympathy with her intentions as well.

The parents will not be unconscious of the attitudes of the staff. They will feel them and be forced to attempt to ignore them if they are not in harmony with their own. But this is a great disappointment and an added task, for the parents know very well that this need not be so. An experience so basic to what it means to be human can be participated in by everyone, each in his own way and according to his own contribution to it. And here the nurse and doctor have much to offer, for they are also flesh and blood. They can also participate in the spiritual value of the experience, so that it becomes their own as well as the parents'. It will mean a personal relation to the parents, but such relations always depend upon what persons share together. If they value the experience as the parents do, they have already established the basis of such communion.

Sincerely,
DAVID D.

Michael

■■■

Dear Mrs. Bing:

Happy Halloween! It's a boy!! All eight pounds of him. Having expected "him" early in October (not the very last day) we attended two complete courses; so perhaps we were more practiced, so to say, but—it was beautiful. Only six hours from the moment I thought I might just have had a slight contraction to the moment of that warm, wet, long-awaited release of life. (I thought it was amazingly easy since it was my first pregnancy and my prior knowledge of childbirth was inferior even to Marjorie Karmel's course at Bryn Mawr—since I only went to City College!)

But seriously . . .

The contractions started at 10:19 and they were so mild I didn't call the doctor till 12:45. But by then they were regular—seven minutes apart. No special breathing was necessary, since by merely relaxing my body (and mind—that's important, since I later learned how easily my imagination runs away with me) I was feeling so calm we decided to walk a few blocks in the sunshine to the bus stop rather than take a cab. I noticed my body responded to a much slower rhythmical pattern of walking, and as long as I didn't fight it there was no pain (this proved true throughout).

On arriving at the hospital, I called the doctor and he advised rushing me to the labor room since the contractions that still seemed merely a "different mild" sensation were three minutes apart. I suppose, since I imagined all first labors to be 13 hours long, I perceived these contractions as slight "preliminaries."

In the labor room was everything I expected, having previously made a tour so that psychologically I was relaxed—the physical conditions were anticipated beforehand.

From 1:30 to 2:30 I was alone, very able to relax my body and use the first breathing technique for these mild three-minute contractions.

By the time my husband joined me, the contractions were increasing in intensity and until three o'clock there was no trouble. In retrospect, I see clearly what was wrong and how next time I might correct it: I had been emphasizing "breathing" over "relaxation" in our trial runs at home, and I seriously underestimated the supreme importance of coordinating a breathing technique for *total* relaxation at the time of a strong contraction. As we had not foreseen the need to practice this breathing in an utterly relaxed state, there were moments of panic. And at the precise moment I panicked and tensed up I lost all control and the breathing was useless, since I was lost to the contraction and my fear of pain. (It is unfortunate that our contemporary civilization completely neglects to educate us in the art of relaxing and controlling the mind.) Whenever my concentration was weakened and I allowed my imagination to anticipate pain, the contraction seemed unbearable and the tension it created multiplied itself. At this point my husband was of greatest help by substituting his reason for my hysteria.

However, I noticed a very interesting thing—there were three times during the worst series of contractions when, for some reason—fatigue or conscious effort or both—my whole body was completely relaxed. At these times I was fully aware of the contraction as a sensation—without the subjective coloration of "pain." I didn't use a breathing technique at these times, for to tear my attention away from the observation of my body would have produced panic—and it was precisely this panicking that made me lose control. Of course, on the positive side, were the frequent times when I was in control and I wasn't victim to the pain. Then it was my husband's encouragement and mere presence that made the difference, though. I don't know if I could have done it alone. (I do think, though, that now, having successfully experienced it and knowing what to expect, I could be just as successful by myself.)

The doctor was wonderful. He seemed to know just what to say at the time it was needed most—he gave me more confidence in myself than I ever could.

In the delivery room I was much more in control and I found the blowing technique, in order not to push, enormously helpful. The breathing was automatic and I quickly found the correct rhythm. With five strong (and surprisingly pleasant) pushes, out came, at 4:30, eight pounds of the most beautiful warm piece of life I or my husband ever saw. The biggest drawback and by far the most unpleasant was, just as I was flushed with the success of victory and an amazing hunger to touch my firstborn, the five hours it took the doctor to sew the stitches; well, at least it seemed like five hours, those ten minutes. Boy, what an uncomfortable thing: I had just "brought forth a life" (and at nineteen and a half years that is quite a profound change) and here was the doctor fooling around for

77

ten minutes at the point. I lost all remembrance of the niceties of civilization and curtly asked the doctor to please hurry up and finish whatever he was doing and stop annoying me!

Feeling exhausted and happy and proud and satisfied and humble ad infinitum and shivering like a leaf, I was wheeled to the recovery room, where I was able to hear the most chilling and horrifying shrieks of uncomprehending agony coming from scared girls all alone in their labor rooms, pleading for help or asking to die. They had no understanding of what was happening to them and nothing with which to control their perception of pain. Their only wish was to be made unconscious and to be deadened to all sensation. I think I cried then more than at any time.

Now back in my room with "the Kid," we'd all (little Michael, Alfred and I) like to thank you for helping to provide us with—well, words aren't enough.

We shall try to spread the news, so maybe some girls will be spared the panic and horror of facing a completely new experience with only fear and misinformation.

I also have to thank you for providing an opportunity for my husband and myself to grow a little closer. I think there's so much more trust now, and we *like* each other a heck of a lot more.

Thanks also for letting me give birth to Michael with awareness and knowledge instead of panic and fear.

Sincerely,

MIRIAM F.

P.S. He's the most beautiful baby I've ever seen!

Martin

●━━━━━━━━━━━━━━━━━━━━━━━━━━━━━━━━━━━━━●

Dear Mrs Bing:

It's taken me a month to find time to type this. So here is my report, and I hope you will enjoy reading it.

I had almost finished taking the course twice, I was one week past my due date, and I had finally decided that the baby wasn't coming until the next week and had made plans for three days of pre-baby activities, when the steady drip, drip of fluid accompanied by contractions began. I said, "This is it—just when I plan things for a few days and forget about waiting for this child, it decides to come." I was sure the labor would take a while and decided to get in one "last meal." It was a picnic meal and sat very well, I thought. However, an hour later, contractions were regular, about nine minutes apart, and I thought then that maybe I shouldn't have eaten.

The contractions continued. A friend had come to dinner and we were to go to a lecture afterward. My husband decided to call the doctor before we left, even though the contractions were not yet five minutes apart. It was our good luck that the doctor had evening hours that day. He said to come on down and we'd see what was happening. So off we went, Tom, Mimi and I (she was amazed at the entire proceeding—so calm in one way and yet so exciting in another). Just in case it was real labor, we took my suitcase.

By 9 P.M. contractions were coming about every five minutes. I started using the slow breathing when necessary. We got to the doctor's office and what do you think? He said I was fully effaced and 3 cm dilated—I was delighted! It was coming at last. I asked did we have time to go to the lecture before checking into the hospital, but taking everything into consideration the doctor decided it would be better not to (the lecture was in New Jersey). My husband had forgotten his antihistamine and I really wanted a shower, and so the doctor said to go home, take care of your business and come back. Mimi was still with us (another stroke of luck, as she lives near the doctor's office). She suggested we come to her place. I showered and Tom got a new prescription filled.

We arrived at the hospital about 11:30 P.M. The clerk kept asking us if we were in a hurry. I said no, I was still using the slow breathing. We got upstairs and were surprised to find out that the staff knew we were "prepared" without even asking us. My goody bag was a giveaway. After I had been given a partial prep the resident examined me. Things had apparently slowed down considerably. I was still only 3 cm dilated, and the contractions were five minutes apart. The resident thought I'd take all night at that rate.

My husband joined me and then things began to pick up again. During the next hour the intervals between contractions decreased to two minutes and by the end of the hour I had started the rapid breathing.

Two hours after his first examination the resident came back to examine me. During those two hours I felt my labor back and front for a while, and then sort of all over.

80

I stopped massaging my abdomen, rested my hands on my chest where my husband could see if they were relaxed. The resident had a funny look on his face. It was shock, I guess, at finding me between 5 and 6 cm dilated, when he didn't really expect any progress. He ran out to call my doctor.

Fifteen minutes later my doctor examined me. I had gone from five to seven cm, and was still comfortably panting.

My doctor and my husband were great. The doctor kept me advised a few minutes *before* each new thing happened. My husband kept me focusing and relaxed. The doctor ruptured the membranes and said, "You will notice a change in the character of the contractions after this, but remember, this is the hardest part. The contractions won't get any stronger than they are now." I noticed a change all right, but I could keep in control, just breathing a little faster than before. I remember that, as the first couple of transition contractions peaked and diminished, I laughed between panting. My husband said, "You're laughing because they won't get any worse." He was right. Now the baby's head was deep in the pelvis. I told the doctor that I had to go to the bathroom. He said, no, I didn't. Then I realized that was what they mean by an urge to push. The next time the urge was stronger—blow, blow, blow for the entire contraction. Another half hour and it would all be over! I was either panting or blowing, but I never did use the pant-blow rhythm effectively. Next time I'm going to really practice this type of breathing! I lost control of about five contractions (not in a row) altogether. My husband got me back and calmed me—I remember him commanding forcefully at times, and I listened.

Up to now there was no medication—no, I take that

back. My husband was there all the time, and if we use medication at times to regain control, I guess that puts him into the category of "medication." I started to push in the labor room and the doctor could see the head in the birth canal. The doctor said the baby had black hair! It was time to go to the delivery room. On the way I chatted on and on, saying, "It's really a baby," in a higher-than-usual voice. When contractions came, I said, "I've got to push!" My husband braced my back and I pushed. My doctor gave me a local and then—whoosh, there came the head, and whoosh, there came the body. "It's a boy, it's a boy (eight pounds, thirteen ounces)." The nurse cleaned off his face and put our son on my chest. Was he heavy! My husband blessed him, and I hugged and kissed my husband.

The process and the moment of birth were so full of awe and wonder and excitement and joy, and we had shared it. I couldn't think of having a baby any other way.

I want to add a postscript: The labor and delivery took eleven hours almost to the minute. The entire process is one of growing physical and emotional stress. It is very hard work!

Sincerely,
Jan M.

Pamela

DEAR MRS. BING:

Well, we had our baby (a splendid little girl).

I emphasize the "we" because my husband felt just as involved as I was. Things went very smoothly and rather quickly. My water broke on the stroke of midnight of my due date and within a half hour the contractions began. I barely had time for that nice warm shower you talked of (and no time to stuff myself with Jello and Tea). At first contractions were erratic, but in an hour's time they were coming sharply and less than five minutes apart. We actually started the fast breathing at home. By 3 A.M. we were in the labor room, and in about an hour we got the go-ahead to push. By some good fortune, I was already 6 cm dilated when I was first examined at the hospital. At 6:45 A.M. the baby was born.

My husband was with me until delivery. I really don't believe it would have been possible for me to have done the breathing and pushing without him. While the labor was relatively short, and we are grateful for that, we sort of missed the preliminary phase of lollipops and talcum powder. It was all work for us from the start. We felt a wonderful sense of accomplishment when it was over, and we firmly believe there can be no more meaningful or healthier way to have a child. The staff at the hospital was cooperative and attentive. Everything was just beautiful. I don't know if the Lamaze method has anything to do with this, but I returned home from the hospital weighing a pound less than when I started my pregnancy. So I thank you, Dr. Lamaze and whoever else is responsible for techniques allowing us to have the unforgettable experience of having our baby together. Now, if there were some way to get a man to take a similar interest in the care and feeding of a newborn . . .

Sincerely,
HARRIET L.

Liza

DEAR MRS. BING:

Having the baby in such a beautiful way was one of the most important experiences of our lives. Bob was high for days, and so was I. He says the change in our lives and his responsibility were much easier to accept and understand emotionally because he was there when Liza was born. Through the birth he was concerned solely with me and then, when it was over, he felt his love and concern grow for Liza, too, and he felt her grow warm in his arms. This may sound pretty corny, but raising children is one of the difficult parts of marriage, and if Lamaze childbirth can help ease a husband's feeling that children are being foisted upon him by some conspiracy, then that should be reason enough for spreading the word.

Since the baby was almost a month late in coming, my husband and I had been out of class for over a month. I was in excellent shape and quite proficient with the breathing techniques, but my husband lost interest in helping me practice toward the end. I consequently practiced less and found my breathing had become less controlled, which was distressing. However, the week before I actually went into labor I practiced a bit more and was almost up to my peak. I should say, I think, that I have had several years of dance, though none in the last four years, can do some yoga and enjoy exercise.

On Thursday night Bob and I went to a movie, an art opening, and then to our favorite pub. I had for several days been experiencing Braxton-Hicks contractions, and at the pub they were more frequent. I joked about being in labor, but by this time neither Bob nor I really believed the baby would ever come and we'd sort of adjusted to me being forever pregnant.

I went to bed about 1:30 A.M. and enjoyed a good sleep until I was awakened about 6 A.M. by frequent "feelings." I thought I might be in labor, but the feelings did not seem to be contractions exactly, and they were certainly not painful. I got up and walked around a little and then tried to time them, but they were so frequent and difficult to detect that I gave up and went back to bed. I woke Bob about 6:30 and asked him if he could please try to time contractions. By this time I was having a little discomfort in my lower back and felt better sitting straight up in bed with my fists dug into my back, though still not doing any regular breathing. This was a funny scene because I'd say "Now Bob" and then again "Now Bob" without ever telling him when they were over. Whatever it was I was having, it was coming so fast that Bob couldn't believe it and refused to show me the time sheet for fear he'd alarm me. By then the discomfort in my back was increasing and I decided I must be one of the unlucky ones with a long back labor ahead of me. I wanted to call the doctor but Bob said it was too early in the morning, and anyway, he said, the contractions couldn't really be two, six, eight, three, etc. minutes apart. I said Mrs. Bing had said they were often irregular, but Bob said not *that* irregular. We finally called at 7:30 A.M. and told the answering service

I wanted to speak to the doctor. By a little after 8 A.M. I still hadn't heard, and in the meantime the contractions were making it quite uncomfortable to walk around and, though still irregular, were sometimes only a minute or two apart. Bob called this time and said I was in labor (I'd neglected to make that clear to the operator) and was put immediately through to the doctor. He described the intervals and said I wasn't in much pain. The doctor said he couldn't believe those were all contractions and that most of it must be just pressure on the rectum and that I was to count the actual contractions, not the pain. I couldn't frankly see the difference, but I dutifully tried to count the bigger ones. I think now that it would have been smarter if I'd talked to the doctor myself because the contractions were becoming more difficult, and, what with a house guest in our two-room apartment and trying to show off to Bob, I hadn't really told him my actual state for several minutes. The doctor said to call back later. I started to get dressed anyway. The idea of waiting a whole lot longer to make it down our four flights of stairs and finding a taxi made me less cavalier. I myself called the doctor the next time, about 8:25, and said I thought I'd really like to get going. He said O.K., that I'd probably be just as comfortable at the hospital anyway. The result was that we didn't get out to find a taxi until the height of the rush hour, and in a light rain on a cold day!

Getting down the stairs was a problem. By this time I simply could not walk more than a few steps without losing control (I thought I could easily keep control with slow deep breathing when sitting down). So I'd rush down one flight, sit down and regain control, then down again until I doubled up and had to sit. Outside, Bob had disappeared, searching for a taxi, so our house guest got my robe

87

out of the suitcase and put it around my legs and I sat on the stoop mostly out of the rain for ten minutes until Bob came. I was still doing the slow breathing but sometimes would pant at the peak of a contraction. I would probably have been more comfortable panting right along at that point, but I supposed that I must have hours and hours to go, since the contractions were much less intense than I'd expected them to be. Going up through the park Bob tried to joke with me but I could only make little grimaces at him; my total concentration was now on the breathing and the contractions.

At the hospital I made it to the admitting office, where they couldn't find our forms and payment record. The lady discerned, however, that I was in no mood to go through the files with her, and when she asked if I wanted a wheelchair to go up to Maternity, I surprised myself by saying "Yes." I still found I was fine until I had to walk, though I was doing mostly early panting. It took ten minutes for them to find a wheelchair. I started getting frustrated with all the waiting. When I finally arrived in Maternity, the intern looked over, saw I was panting and said, "Good, that's the best way," and then left me sitting there. The nurse took me into the room for prepping. The minute I sat down I had the urge to push and yelled out for the nurse and told her to get an intern immediately, that I wanted to be examined. The intern examined me, asked the nurse to make sure my doctor was on his way, and congratulated me, saying I'd done very well at home and was fully dilated and ready to deliver! So everything fell into place. Those were real contractions I'd been experiencing, and now I wasn't even going to get a chance to do all I'd practiced. I got a quick partial prep. The doctor arrived and dashed off to find Bob, who was down in the admitting office trying to get my records straightened

88

out. He, of course, hadn't been allowed to be with me through any of the labor-room drama. By this time there was no space at all between contractions, and I was blowing with all my might. My body pushed a little despite my biggest efforts. And here, for me, was the big challenge: to hold off the birth of the baby till Bob and the doctor could be with me.

I was moved into the delivery room while Bob and the doctor had a quick scrub (Bob came out with his mask on backward). Here the staff went into a comedy routine. I was blowing like crazy when I heard my doctor say, "Oh my God, they've installed the new tables and we haven't had a dry run yet!" Whereupon the doctor, two interns and I don't know how many nurses started trying to adjust the new delivery table. They kept asking if the stirrups were comfortable, and I kept saying I didn't really care, that I'd just like to have the baby please. I suppose this didn't take more than two minutes, but it seemed longer because of the tremendous strain of fighting the urge to push. Finally the doctor said I could give one tiny little push and then to blow some more. He performed a fast episiotomy and let me push once more and out came the baby. Bob, who had been encouraging me during the blowing and propping my shoulders (though I was actually very strong from so short a labor), was the one who said, "It's a girl." And after they cleaned her up a bit (she cried without needing a slap!) and I held her for a few minutes, I gave her to Bob to hold. He held her for ten to fifteen minutes. She was very alert and when she first opened her eyes she looked up at him, and he will never get over the thrill of being with her during her first moments of life in this world.

Sincerely,
SHARON P. S.

Jennifer

DEAR MRS. BING:

Having had one child in the usual method of fear, anxiety, ignorance and pain, I decided there must be a better and more pleasant way. Receptive to new ideas, I listened eagerly as a friend related her thrilling experience with the Lamaze method of childbirth.

I was determined to find a course in New York City that would enlighten me. After some difficulty, I found you, Mrs. Bing, and that became the beginning of a wonderful experience.

For six weeks my husband and I traveled to Manhattan for a stimulating, interesting and purely enjoyable evening with you and the other couples whom we met in our class. For me the classes opened up a world previously closed and intentionally avoided. For the first time in my life I was truly interested in finding out about birth, in facing up to its intricacies, and in exposing myself and my modesties to the realities of a very basic part of human existence without fear and repulsion. This was really new for me and extremely therapeutic. I became very excited about having a baby and being awake during its birth, and I waited happily for the occasion to present itself.

On December 4th at 5:30 A.M. I was awakened by my first real contraction. For the next half hour I waited with excitement for each contraction. They were clearly coming at intervals of four to five minutes. My next step was to start packing, and I ran around the apartment in a disorganized fashion throwing things into a suitcase.

My husband awoke in the darkness of a rainy early morning to inquire what was going on. I told him about the contractions, we called the doctor, arranged for the older child to be taken care of, finished packing, filled our goody bag, not forgetting essential nourishment for my husband. By 6:45 we were on our way to the hospital.

In the car I had the first opportunity to relax and practice the first breathing technique. I immediately felt better. By 7 A.M. we found ourselves at the admitting desk, where the clerk politely waited while I "breathed" through my contractions.

I was then taken upstairs to the labor room and my husband had to wait until I was prepped and he could join me again. The hospital did not really like husbands in the labor room, and my husband was asked again and again to step out, so that we spent little time uninterrupted together.

Luckily, the time in the labor room was blissfully short. My labor progressed quickly and I soon switched to the fast breathing technique. When my husband was with me, he was encouraging and firm in his directions. He quickly pointed out how I could improve my position, he kept me to a good rhythm in breathing and he gently wiped my brow with the washcloth.

The doctor had suggested earlier that I accept a small amount of Demerol, and had promised that it would not put me out, but just take the edge off. I believe it did just that. I know it helped me to relax between contractions, and I felt blissfully sleepy and calm during the intervals of rest.

The breathing techniques were the mainstay of my comfort and control and most of all my confidence.

By 9:30 A.M. my doctor told me that he would take me to the delivery room. I had, just prior to that, switched to the third breathing exercise. My husband unfortunately was then asked to leave me and wait downstairs. I knew he felt very bad about having to leave, just as I did, and I vowed that next time he would stay with me in the delivery room, even if we have to change doctor and hospital.

My legs were put into stirrups and I asked that the mirror be adjusted so that I could watch my baby being born. The staff seemed to be less harried and more cheerful in the delivery room, or was that a projection of my own feelings now?

The anesthesiologist stood by most of the time encouraging me to take something. But I told him no, and my doctor informed him to leave me alone and that "If she wants something, she'll let us know."

I worked very hard and pushed and pushed . . . and then as the baby's head was about to appear, I looked into the mirror and I saw my child being born, and it almost seemed as if the drama taking place in the mirror was somehow not really related to me. Then they told me it was a girl, and I was suddenly ecstatic. She really was ugly, but I screamed, "My girl, my beautiful girl!"

They held her up for me to see, umbilical cord and all.

By 10:20 A.M. I was in the recovery room, a little sleepy, but feeling great otherwise. After all, I had seen my daughter being born! I knew then that there really is no other way to have a baby.

Sincerely,
SANDRA F.

Deborah

Dear Mrs. Bing:

All I can say is thank you.

And here is my report:

It was Sunday, January 5th, when my contractions began. They were rather mild. I had been expecting something to happen because I had had abdominal cramps the previous two nights. Before waking my husband I decided to time my contractions. I went to the living room, sat in our rocker, drank hot, sweet tea, and did the slow breathing exercise. At 9:30 A.M., after timing the contractions for two hours, I called the doctor. The contractions were seven minutes apart and the doctor said to come to the hospital without rushing. Then I awoke my husband.

I could tell that my husband was happy. I think that he was beginning to think that there wasn't going to be a baby after all. We both began getting ready and were very calm about the whole situation. I packed fruit, candy and cookies for my husband, so that he could have something to eat, and made sure that our goody bag had everything in it. My husband packed our personal telephone directory in his briefcase so that he could call everyone right from the hospital. He was bouncing around the house, as happy as could be that morning!

It was very cold out as we drove to the hospital, and I couldn't believe that the time had really come! I did my slow breathing and kept timing my contractions. Then I began to get worried because they weren't getting any closer together. I kept thinking they'd send me home once I got to the hospital, and I didn't want to have to go back home—I wanted to have my baby.

We arrived at the hospital around 11:30 A.M. When we went into the labor room, around 12:45 P.M., my contractions were still no closer together. After the doctor's examination, we found out that the baby was in a breech position. I was worried, but the doctor said I should do everything just as I had been instructed. Then I felt more confident. I was given some pills to speed along my contractions. Around 2:30 P.M. I started the panting breathing. I found the rubbing of my abdomen very helpful and relaxing. The lollipop was also a great help, even though the nurse frowned upon it.

Around 3:30 P.M. my contractions were getting closer together and continued in this way until I had hardly any time at all between contractions. I was really concentrating now (I used the light on the ceiling as a focal point) and I grabbed for the lollipop whenever I could. The only thing that irritated me was when the nurse pressed on my abdomen during a contraction to feel the strength of it. It made things very uncomfortable.

I never used the third breathing technique, because the doctor came in at this time and told me I could start pushing. I found this pushing stage (in the labor room) the easiest and most relieving. My husband was the greatest help at this point, and with his encouragement I felt I was really doing a good job. My husband was even more help at this point than the nurse because he knew at what

94

point to hold my head for me. I did have a rest between each of these contractions and it felt great to throw my head back and pant slowly.

I pushed in the labor room about forty minutes, after which I had a small shot of Demerol before going into the delivery room. I pushed the baby's bottom out. What a release I felt! I was given an anesthetic, though, when the head was delivered. When I awoke in the recovery room I found I had a baby girl—twenty-two inches, seven pounds, ten ounces. My husband had seen her born!

Sincerely,

Joan J.

Matthew Roy

●●●

DEAR MRS. BING:

As you requested, I am writing a recap of what was a delightful experience.

Matthew Roy, eight kicking pounds and twenty-two inches long, was delivered just three and a half hours after my first uterine contraction.

My due date was Tuesday, February 18. The preceding week, during the worst snowstorm of the winter, I had many hours of false labor, ending (wouldn't you know?) with the end of the snow.

On Saturday, three days early, I had what I thought was the first sign of the bloody show, but it was not enough to really tell.

I awoke Monday morning at 7 A.M. to find the membranes had ruptured one day early. I waited until 9 A.M. to call the doctor's office, and his nurse advised me to leave immediately for the hospital, as it is an hour's drive from our home. However, I was not having any contractions and, as my husband works in the evenings, I let him sleep until nearly 10 A.M., while I did some minor chores around the house. After a leisurely departure, we arrived at the hospital at 12:30 P.M., where I was immediately taken to an admitting bed until I could be examined by the resident physician. My husband was allowed to join me by 1 P.M.

My first contractions started about 2 P.M., although they were painless and required no breathing exercises. The resident physician examined me at 2:30 P.M. after I had experienced only three contractions worth doing preliminary breathing. He said I was only 1 cm dilated and ordered an enema be given to me. As is my doctor's practice, I was not prepped (one indignity less).

Since my membranes had already ruptured and I was flowing copiously, the enema was given to me in bed, and I was left alone with the impossible task of using a bed pan while enclosed in a curtained-off area in the mainstream of traffic. The nurse caught me trying to use the bed pan off the side of the bed, as you suggested, and I was ordered back into bed. Somehow I survived the ordeal, but it was humiliating.

The enema seemed to speed up the contractions, which started coming about every two minutes and lasting about forty-five seconds. My husband was now with me and was timing the contractions as I did the preliminary breathing. The contractions remained at two-minute intervals and did not change much in intensity.

At 3:30 P.M. I was moved to the labor room. There the contractions again began to fluctuate in length and intensity. They would come in series of three: a 45-second one, 30-second interval, 90-second contraction, 30-second interval, 45-second contraction. Then the next series would be the reverse: 90-second, 45-second, 90-second, with 30-second intervals. Each series of three seemed to be delayed by a 60-second interval. It was somewhat confusing. I continued with the preliminary breathing until 4 P.M., perplexed by the irregularity. The contractions began to hurt around 4:30 P.M. and I switched to the accelerated breathing. About this time the resident physician again examined me and said I was 4 cm dilated. I groaned at the thought of not even being halfway there.

At 5 P.M. I began to feel a great deal of pain, although the contractions were still irregular. My husband had given up trying to time them because it seemed like a useless proposition, and I was beginning to feel discouraged because the accelerated breathing was not enough at this point and I still had 6 cm to go. I had no urge to push and began to feel that if I had hours more of this type of pain I would not be able to last.

The nurse had twice asked me if I wanted to take a little Demerol, and she put the question in such a way that I began to feel a little guilty for refusing medication. She said that it was bad for the baby if I was tensing up, and the Demerol would help me relax and stop fighting. I certainly did not feel I was fighting, but the thought of many more hours at equal or greater intensity was discouraging. My mood, at this point, was at a low, and I should have remembered from my lessons that being irritable and in a bad mood was one of the symptoms of having reached the transitional phase. After discussing the situation with my husband, I decided to take 50 cc's of Demerol. I told the nurse, but before she could bring it my doctor arrived, examined me and told me that I was fully dilated and had passed right through transition. We were all amazed that I had not had the desire to push. Knowing that I was so close to delivery, my mood and outlook changed, and I did not take the drug. When I began to push, I felt complete relief. True, it was hard work, but it was far preferable to the contractions I had been experiencing.

Somehow I had dilated 6 cm in less than half an hour.

I pushed for another half hour, during which I was moved to the delivery room. At the very end, the doctor asked my permission to perform an episiotomy, which he had agreed earlier would only be done if necessary. He made the cut after giving me a needle. It was over in a moment. I tried three more pushing contractions and could not seem to expel the child. During the contraction, I had to take a new breath four times, but the last two times were never effective; I did not manage to hold my breath for pushing but always ended up with straining in my throat and expelling air in a gurgling sound.

At this point the doctor said that it just was not working even though I was so close, and that he would have to use forceps to deliver the baby. He then inserted the forceps, and, as I watched, he gave a little tug with the next contraction. At 5:34 P.M. out came an eight-pound kicking boy. The afterbirth was delivered before the next contraction and before I could ask the doctor to wait, but I was too excited and too busy asking my husband whether he liked the child. Within minutes I was sewn up and given my son to nurse while still on the delivery table.

Throughout the whole labor my husband attended to me with lollipops, washcloths and unlimited encouragement. He had not intended to come into the delivery room, but when the time came he felt that he just could not leave me after coming so far with me. He feels today that our son was delivered by both of us and tells our friends that it was the most remarkable and intense thing he was ever allowed to participate in. In fact, he is more prone to discuss our labor than I am.

I was in the rooming-in section of the hospital and recovered fast enough to be discharged in four days. I was up and around the next morning and felt nothing but a sore bottom. I have had no problem with stitches, and no other pains or aftereffects.

Now, twelve days after the delivery, our boy is two ounces over his eight-pound birth weight and has grown half an inch. I feel certain that the total lack of drugs in both our systems has made him the active and healthy baby he is.

Thank you again for your course and advice. I certainly intend to use the psychoprophylactic method for my future children.

Sincerely,
SUSAN J.

Stephen

DEAR MRS. BING:

My son arrived three weeks late on a cold January afternoon, just when I had begun to doubt if there really was a baby after all. By that time I was thoroughly sick of the Jello I kept making to eat in early labor and quite frustrated because I had been having strong, irregular contractions for the past two weeks which never went into actual labor. Consequently I wasn't too excited when I again awoke with irregular contractions at 3 A.M. and managed to drop off to sleep between them. However, by 4:30 A.M., they suddenly became stronger and were about five minutes apart. I woke my husband, who, in spite of earlier promises to be calm, followed me around the house holding my coat (I was still in my nightgown), insisting that we call my doctor and leave immediately for the hospital. By 5:45 A.M. the contractions were still coming steadily at four minutes apart, and on my doctor's instructions we left for the hospital. I was now doing the first breathing and found it much easier to sit than to stand.

My first examination was by a staff physician who pronounced me 4 cm dilated and muttered a few not-too-encouraging words about the baby's largeness and my smallness and long labors. He also spotted my Lamaze bag and announced in no uncertain terms that peppermint sticks to suck on were absolutely taboo—apparently he considered this eating.

Forty-five minutes later I was examined by my doctor's associate (my doctor's car had broken down) and I learned that everything was fine and I was already between 5 and 6 cm dilated. I was moved from the prep room to the labor floor and reunited with my husband. We were joined by three student nurses who were fascinated by the Lamaze breathing—they were marvelously friendly and helpful and nearly fell over each other trying to make me comfortable with Chapstick, back rubs and cold washcloths on my face. We put my husband in charge of the stopwatch. By now the contractions were exactly three minutes apart, and I shifted without thinking to the accelerated breathing. Edward would announce, "There's one coming in ten seconds," and we would all get ready; during the intervals the five of us chatted as if we were all old friends. I was very lucky that there were no other women in labor at the time and I had this extra attention.

At 9:30 my doctor arrived and told me I was still dilated at 6 cm. He then broke the membranes and almost immediately I experienced much stronger contractions, which I felt a little threatened by until I got used to them, and then I managed quite well. For some reason I still don't understand, I began feeling a tightening low in the pelvic area about fifteen seconds before the uterus got hard. Toward 11 A.M. I began to notice that I was also still feeling the contractions low in the back after the nurses felt the uterus had relaxed. So I changed from lying at a slight angle to sitting straight up. As soon as I did this the problem was eliminated and I felt completely in control and very relaxed. About fifteen minutes later, how-

102

ever, a hot flush and a wave of nausea swept over me and I vomited several times. The contractions were now intense, coming every minute and fifteen seconds and were felt mostly in the lower back. I was very sure that I was in the transition phase and started the pant-and-blow breathing. I was utterly crushed when the examining resident said that I was still 6 cm dilated and nowhere near the transition. (I wish I had realized that two doctors can give entirely different evaluations of one's progress. As my doctor explained later: "One man's six cm is another man's eight cm.") At any rate, this resident insisted that I lie flat on my back and proceeded to give me a lecture on being grateful for having such an easy time. I suppose he had a point, but I didn't feel like hearing it just then! Soon the contractions were coming every thirty seconds, and shortly after that, one just seemed to blend into the next in unpredictable waves. I found it quite difficult to breathe and stay on top and found myself racing along behind the contractions. I now think this problem could have been eased somewhat if I had been allowed to sit up, as a change in position had worked so well in the earlier stages.

All during this time there were from six to eight people around my bed, listening to the fetal heartbeat, wiping my face, trying to take my temperature, pressing against my back—and all giving me advice. With all this activity, my husband was temporarily pushed into the background and didn't realize I was having difficulty coordinating the breathing with the waves of the contractions. (I had by now simply stopped talking to anyone.)

The next examination revealed that I had dilated to 9 cm. My doctor gave me a small dose of Demerol to help me relax, and the contractions raced on the same way for the next half hour. At 12:40 P.M. they began to ease and were more clearly defined again. My doctor then said I could push as soon as I felt the urge. I waited a while and felt nothing, so I asked a nurse if I could push anyway. She said, "No, it would only waste your energy." This didn't make any sense to me, so I decided to keep quiet and start pushing anyway. I proceeded a little cautiously at first, but as soon as I pushed with all my strength, I felt a great relief and absolutely no pain.

I can hardly describe the tremendous change in my feeling at that point. I was exhilarated by the discovery that this didn't hurt at all and felt so full of strength and confidence that I could have gone on for hours. I could now smile at everyone and make jokes between contractions. I could also sense the excitement in the room as they watched the baby's head come more and more into view, and I wanted to hug my husband for all his encouragement and praise.

We all moved down the hall to the delivery room at 12:45 P.M. (the three student nurses were determinedly sticking it out even though they were now off duty). Once into position on the delivery table, I had pushed halfway through another contraction when suddenly a rubber mask was slapped over my face and a soothing voice urged me to "inhale and all the pain will go away." This was the last thing in the world I wanted or needed, and the well-meaning anesthesiologist meekly retreated. I was so completely involved in the pushing, I could hardly bear to stop to take another breath.

Before I knew it, it was 1:08 P.M., and I felt something wet and wiggling on my thigh, and the doctor held up a perfect baby boy. I glanced happily from the baby to my husband, and the look of wonder and pride on his face completely erased any doubts I might have had that this was really a marvelous way to have a baby.

I was even more convinced of this as I became acquainted with some of the other new mothers in the hospital. The majority looked back on their childbirth experience as something of a nightmare they definitely would rather forget—as an experience they'd had to endure all alone, as an experience their husbands ("You know how men are") simply could not understand or help them with in any way. I realized then how much it meant to me to have experienced the birth of my baby as the thrilling and satisfying event it should be, and I was happy too for the tremendous closeness it brought to my husband and me.

Sincerely,
CAROLINE W.

Jason

●━━●

DEAR MRS. BING:

Here is my report on Jason's birth:

On Tuesday morning I saw my doctor for my regular visit. He had given me a due date for November 21st and here it was only October 29th; therefore I didn't expect to hear him tell me I was already 4 cm dilated. He said that I could have my baby that day or in a week.

I then recalled that I had been having Braxton-Hicks contractions for a few days. The next Monday morning I attended my fourth Lamaze class, where I learned the pushing technique. I felt fine, with no discomfort, and I didn't associate the events of the previous few days as being perhaps early labor. On Monday night I practiced the pushing technique with my husband. On Tuesday I felt fine, though somewhat tired, and I slept almost all afternoon.

At about 2 A.M. the following morning, while I was fast asleep, the membranes ruptured. Paul called the doctor and he told us to go straight to the hospital. We could hardly believe this was the day we had been waiting for so long. I felt great—no discomfort other than wetness. Paul was nervous but managed wonderfully. I never had time to pack my suitcase, so I just grabbed the goody bag and your book, and we drove the twenty minutes to the hospital. We felt like two actors who had been re-hearsing for our first play and were now eagerly looking forward to see how our performance would go.

After the preliminary admitting procedure, Paul waited downstairs while I was prepared for labor. I was a little bit disappointed when I found out I was still only 4 cm dilated, but I recalled the doctor telling me that once I went into active labor it would go very quickly. I still had no contractions. After the enema I began to have very slight contractions, so slight that I couldn't feel them rise or fall—only when they were at the peak. I still felt great.

Paul joined me in the labor room around 3 A.M. and we found that we had a nurse who was trained in the Lamaze method. This proved a tremendous help, mostly because I hadn't had time to practice my breathing as the baby was over three weeks early, and also because I could not feel the contractions coming on. She put her hand on my uterus and told me when to commence my breathing. Then she reviewed with Paul and me the proper technique. Most of the time she breathed with me and I used her as my point of concentration. Paul counted off the time, as he had done during our practice sessions. Paul also told me when I was tensing my muscles and helped me relax my arms and legs. He was a tremendous help to my relaxation and general behavior. With him by my side I had strong confidence that everything would be fine. His presence was extremely necessary for me.

My bed was at a slant, and I was sort of sitting up. As the sun was rising, I decided to start the first breathing technique. The contractions were about two minutes apart, but were so slight that I continued to use the first breathing technique. I massaged my abdomen but felt no need for talc or lollipops.

After about one hour the contractions became stronger

107

and I switched to the second breathing exercise. It was now about 7 A.M. I felt no great discomfort and I was amazed at how great everything was going.

At about 8 A.M. things started to happen. My doctor examined me and found me to be 8 cm dilated. I then felt a need for transitional breathing. I began to get excited, knowing that my baby would be born soon. However, I breathed automatically, as I had been trained to do, and felt in control of the situation.

Soon the doctor told me to start pushing. It was all so sudden—I was overwhelmed with excitement. I didn't feel the urge to push, but I tried to bear down nevertheless. Then the doctor said, "Into the delivery room," and I was surprised that I felt so wonderful.

My husband was right by my side in the delivery room. At this time my first problem occurred. I didn't feel any urge to push—not the slightest. I had had just one demonstration in pushing and had not had time to practice it at home. Therefore I had no control over the muscles that would be involved in pushing my baby out. Here I realized completely the difference proper training can make, for I felt that if I had learned to control these muscles, I would have been able to push effectively even though I didn't feel the urge to do so.

With the nurses and my husband giving the commands, I tried my hardest to push when the doctor said to do so —but to no avail. I could feel my baby moving, but I just couldn't work my muscles. Therefore my doctor had to manually help push my baby out. There was no discomfort, only extreme excitement. I believe it took four pushes by the doctor, and my baby was born.

I saw the doctor hold him upside down and say, "It's a boy!" and then he laid him on my abdomen. That was the most fantastic moment of my life—to look into the face of my first baby. I then felt as though I was being born also—I had entered the world of motherhood. As a family, we were off to the best start possible.

I'm sure the most intimate and precious emotions my husband and I felt are shared by other couples whose babies are born with the Lamaze method.

Thank you so much, Mrs. Bing, for enabling us to have Jason born the way we intended.

We look forward to seeing you when we expect our second baby.

Sincerely,
DIANA K.

Shana

DEAR MRS. BING:

My first interest in the Lamaze method was generated by a somewhat chickenhearted attitude toward childbirth. I was, in the dreadful terminology of pregnancy manuals, an elderly primapara, thirty-four years old; I wondered if my ancient pelvic muscles would cooperate to bring forth a child. Sometime during the eighth month of pregnancy the fear hit me.

"My God, there's a big baby in there—how on earth am I ever going to get it out?"

To learn that I could do something active and positive to help myself during labor instead of being a victim, that I could not only avoid pain but make this birth a beautiful experience for me and my husband, sold me on the Lamaze technique.

I got plenty of discouragement from those women who either could not or would not experience a prepared birth. Their comments ranged from the humorous to the psychoanalytic to the downright malicious. What surprised me most was the rabid quality of their opinions, as though approaches to childbirth were in the same sensitive area as politics and religion.

"Don't tell me it doesn't hurt . . . I *know*!"

"What are you trying to prove?"

"Next time I want to be put out with the first pain and wake up when the hairdresser arrives."

"I think natural childbirth is wildly masochistic!"

"How can you allow your husband to see you suffer so horribly—are you trying to punish him?"

Strangely enough, most of these negative comments came from women who had had anesthetics. If all those painkillers are so great, I thought, how come these mothers had such anguished recollections? Not one of them had had either a prepared birth or the emotional support of a trained husband. It took a lot of reading on psychoprophylaxis and several Lamaze classes for me to overcome the grisly myths of all my early conditioning. But after the third class, I knew—and my husband knew—that there was simply no other way for me to have a baby.

11:45 p.m. First contraction. I suspected this might be just another session of mild "menstrual cramps" which I had been having for several nights, so I awoke my husband with an apologetic poke to tell him that I might possibly be in labor. He shot out of bed, got the stopwatch in hand, and we both waited. Exactly twelve minutes later, another cramp, followed by a series of menstrual sensations spaced just seven minutes apart. Each one lasted forty-five seconds. Although I was terribly excited about the possibility of being in labor, I just couldn't believe my husband's assurance that this was really "it."

12:45 a.m. After another hour of regular seven- to eight-minute contractions, I finally agreed to "disturb" the doctor. My husband, placing his hand on my belly, could now tell me when a contraction was coming. He said that he could feel the uterus drawing itself up into a tight, hard mass, a few seconds ahead of time. So this convinced me.

111

I told a sleepy doctor that I might be in labor, and could I have a stiff drink to celebrate. He said yes, I was, and yes, I could, and to come to the hospital when the contractions were spaced about five minutes apart. Right after I hung up I had a fierce attack of diarrhea. We spent the next few hours sipping vodka, playing with the stopwatch and calling all our friends in California, where it was a civilized three hours earlier. We were just too excited and happy to sleep.

3:00 A.M. Contractions irregularly five to six minutes apart and forty-five seconds in duration. I began to pack my bag and get dressed. We both spent a ludicrous amount of time fussing about what we were going to wear. We checked all the objects in our Lamaze bag three times. We had been practicing seven weeks for this miraculous evening, and now that it was here it didn't seem real. I couldn't believe that something this much fun could really be labor. There was no need to use any of the breathing techniques as yet.

4:30 A.M. No red tape at the hospital. After a brief admission procedure, we were led to what was to be my permanent home. I got into bed, armed with my lollipops. My husband went down for coffee. A resident doctor examined me and told me I was 85 percent effaced and 2 cm dilated. Lovely young nurses floated in every fifteen minutes with all the trappings of their trade: blood-pressure machines, thermometers, etc. Thanks to the 1:30 A.M. attack of diarrhea, I didn't have to get an enema, and since my doctor didn't believe in prepping, I was also spared this indignity. In spite of all the warnings in class, we had gone to the hospital too early and sleep was impossible; my husband's chair was slippery and badly angled for him to snooze. Each time he started to doze off, he would slide downward. I was too fascinated with the sensation of my contractions. So we read magazines and made small talk until 8:30 in the morning when the obstetrician came in to examine me.

8:30 A.M. Contractions four to five minutes apart, lasting a minute. My doctor's examination was the first real moment of discomfort. It was a miserable sensation, that long probing and pushing around in me during a contraction. He reported that I was now 3 cm dilated (only one centimeter of progress in 4 hours!) and that the head, although nicely engaged, was not yet in proper position to do its work of pressing against the cervix. This was responsible for both the slow dilation and discomfort of the examination. He predicted the baby would probably not come till late afternoon. When he mentioned my going up to the labor room I begged him to postpone it as long as possible. I dreaded being placed within earshot of some bellowing female.

9:00 A.M. Contractions about three and a half to four minutes apart. I tried sitting up in a chair, which I found most comfortable; but almost immediately a nurse came in and shooed me back into bed—hospital policy. Somehow, sitting up in bed was not as satisfactory; it placed too much pressure on my rectum. My husband and I experimented with rolling the back and knee sections of the bed to different levels until we found the most comfortable angles, and I spent the remainder of my labor in variations of this position. Without having to think about it, I began the slow chest breathing and abdominal massage. We continued to time the contractions just because it gave us something to do. Some amusing social distraction was provided by friends calling up to ask if it was a boy or a girl.

10:45 A.M. Contractions gaining force, averaging three to three and a half minutes apart, and lasting for a full minute or more. The chest breathing no longer seemed quite sufficient, so I began a very shallow, fast panting in 4-4 rhythm. This proved fully effective in keeping me on top of each wave.

11:45 A.M. After twelve hours of labor, my doctor's associate came in to subject me to another grinding, twisting examination.

"You are doing just beautifully," he said.

"How far am I dilated?"

"Three centimeters."

"Three centimeters!" I said. "My God, no progress at all—I was three centimeters three damned hours ago!"

He gave me some cheery talk about the head having worked itself into the proper position against the cervix; he said that labor would become more effective very soon and that I would have to be taken up to the labor room presently. The contractions had increased in intensity by about 10 percent, but I was still quite able to experience them as interesting muscular sensations.

12:45 P.M. I was shifted into a stretcher and taken up to the labor rooms. Although each of these little cubicles was private, there was no soundproofing. No sooner had I gotten settled on my leather bed than two women down the hall embarked on a strident duet of howling and moaning. My husband, in an attempt to drown out our labormates, turned on the electric fan. Although this put us both in an awful draft, it was well worth the chill not to have to listen to the caterwauling. Strangely enough, I felt no sympathy for those women; the flamboyant stupidity of their behavior infuriated me.

1:00 P.M. Contractions now two and a half minutes

apart, lasting sixty to ninety seconds. Now I no longer wanted to be left alone. My husband left for the bathroom. He was only gone ten minutes, but to me it seemed like an hour. The doctor arrived, examined me and reported only ½ cm progress in dilation. Since I had been laboring for about thirteen hours with not much to show for it, he now decided to rupture the membranes. He had not wanted to do this earlier, as it would have put too much uterine pressure on an undilated cervix. I huffed and puffed something fierce during the water-breaking maneuver, which was followed by a tremendous gush of warm water, but no immediate acceleration of labor. I was still panting lightly in 4-4 time, not tired at all, and in full control. With each contraction, another gush of water spurted forth. The angels of mercy gave me clean bedding under my bottom each time they came to check the fetal heartbeat—about every fifteen minutes.

2:30 P.M. Contractions two to two and a half minutes apart lasting seventy-five to ninety seconds. The doctor's examination showed me to be 4 cm dilated. He complimented me on the forcible nature of my contractions, and assured me I would make more progress in the next two hours than I had done all day. My husband was most helpful in reminding me to take a "cleansing breath" before and after each session of panting. Contractions were coming on like gangbusters, and sometimes, in my eagerness to catch them in time, I would omit that first deep breath. They would peak almost immediately, stay at full intensity for forty-five seconds, and take another forty-five seconds to die down.

3:00 P.M. My doctor suggested 50 mg of Demerol—just to relax. I didn't feel very tense, but my husband and I were working hard by now. I had become a sort of human machine, responding to the stopwatch, panting in time and relaxing. At first I argued with the doctor, assuring him that I could go on for hours without taking any drugs, but he convinced me that a tiny dose of Demerol would be helpful to our efforts. It wasn't! It did nothing to relieve the powerful contractions—it merely fouled up my ability to concentrate, to "catch" each contraction before it caught me. I felt very much like a drunk trying to walk a straight line.

3:30 P.M. For the first time in sixteen hours of labor, I was in pain—not suffering, not frightened, but nevertheless in pain. A fantastic sensation—powerful, pulling cramps starting in the lower belly and radiating around to the back. The old cliché, "Doctor, it grips me like a vise," floated in my mind. Contractions were coming every one and a half to two and a half minutes, lasting one to two minutes. My husband hung a bright red washcloth up on the wall for me to concentrate on. His love and support were ten times more effective than any drug; as soon as I was able to work with him, the pain receded.

4 P.M. Contractions coming every minute and lasting forty-five seconds. Examination showed 4½ centimeters of dilation—head pressing powerfully against the cervix. I was given some oval white hormone pellets to slip under my upper lip. The doctor told me these were to accelerate labor.

4:40 P.M. Examination: dilated to 5 cm. Contractions becoming formidable—almost impossible to stay calm and relaxed. Even though I knew the small dose of Demerol I'd had earlier hadn't helped a bit, I heard myself asking for "a little something to take the edge off." The doctor told me I would be in the expulsive stage before any drug had a chance to take effect. Moments later I was drenched

116

with sweat; my arms and legs began to jerk and tremble uncontrollably. Twice I wanted to vomit but was unable to produce anything but a loud dry burp. So this was it —transition. It was not so much painful as it was terrifying. Nothing—no class or movie or medical description —could have prepared me for the titanic force of those last contractions.

4:55 P.M. Suddenly, the urge to push! I wanted to push more than anything in the world. My husband dashed into the hallway to nab the doctor; he found me 8½ centimeters dilated. I blew out constantly to counter the violent urge to push.

5:05 P.M. Given permission to push—great confusion. I had been working so hard *not* to push that I suddenly forgot how to do it. With three sloppy, badly executed pushes, I thought I felt my baby's head hit the pelvic floor—thump!

5:15 P.M. I was hurried into the delivery room, shifted onto a leather-and-steel monstrosity of a table and draped with sheets. The doctor barely had time to scrub. Now I was pushing fit to bust; it was the most strenuous effort of my life. My husband held my back up with each push; it was just as though we were pushing the baby out together. What a wonderful comfort it was to see his face and feel him hold me. On the fifth push, the head crowned, and I was told to pant. This was the second time I almost chickened out. I heard myself mutter, "Give me a little whiff of something." Two anesthesiologists wheeled over evil-looking green gas tanks. My husband and doctor chased them away. We were just too close to victory to give in now. I heard the doctor making an incision; it sounded like heavy shears cutting canvas. There was no pain. Then the magic words came: "Only one more push!"

117

5:29 P.M. I pushed until I felt I couldn't push any more. I pushed with every muscle in my body. I heard a little cry, and then I felt her slip out of me—twenty inches of beautiful, warm, wet baby girl! Someone put her on my stomach, and after looking her over quickly, I asked everyone in the room if I could kiss my husband. Although I am madly in love with that man, never before had I loved him quite this much. To me he was the strongest, most masculine man in the world. He had given birth to her as much as I had; it was beautiful.

6:15 P.M. I was taken back to my room, where my husband was waiting for me with a bottle of iced champagne. I suggest that some of this festive bubbly stuff be included in every Lamaze bag. After twenty-two hours without food, I was ravenous! I ordered everything on the hospital menu, including a big gooey dessert. While waiting for our little girl to be brought in, I wandered around the room (later I learned that this was strictly *verboten*), called all my close friends and guzzled the remaining champagne.

I cannot remember ever having been happier. Now we knew what life was all about! Although the last two hours of my labor had been far from painless, I had not suffered. The definition of suffering does not include the sense of exhilaration and accomplishment that comes from having witnessed a miracle.

Sincerely,
NANCY F. M.

118

Jordan

●━━━━━━━━━━━━━━━━━━━━━━━━━━━━━━━●

Dear Mrs. Bing:

My baby was born two days ago and today he and my wife are together with us again. That in itself may not seem like a tremendous accomplishment, but the circumstances surrounding the birth and their quick return home are quite exciting.

Eric, our first child, was born two and one-half years ago under circumstances that were amazingly normal. Normal in the sense that they were common, rather than natural. My wife had the usual pain and drug treatment for labor and delivery. I was ushered out so as not to be in the way of the professionals performing their specialty. (It was not until recently that I found out how poorly they did that.) My wife had the usual slow recovery period back to normal and the usual poor images of her experience.

The experience which we have recently shared was substantially different. During labor, although much of the time there was nothing much for me to do, I felt that I was needed and a help. If only to give certain reminders or run errands or give comfort, I was there. Near the end of the first stage of labor Margie began to lose control and was having a problem with her contractions and control

119

and she asked me to get the doctor to give her some medication. The doctor came in to administer it but examined her and told her that she was almost fully dilated. At this point the nurse told me to get ready to be with Margie in the delivery room. Upon hearing this, Margie seemed to forget all pain and an unbelievable transformation took place. The problems that she had been having moments before vanished, and she became excited and cheerful. It certainly made me feel great to know that just the thought of my presence in the delivery room could create such a difference. The rest was accomplished without difficulty.

I had seen a film on the process of childbirth and so was prepared for the physical events that I witnessed in the delivery room. But the emotional thrill of seeing my child being born and especially experiencing the event together with my wife is a feeling that I doubt can be approximated in any other way. You sit and watch and try to express what you are seeing in words like "fantastic" and "unbelievable" and find that words are so inadequate to describe the feelings that are taking place in yourself, flowing between you and your wife with every touch.

My wife's recovery was a very surprising situation to me. After Eric was born there had been a slow recovery back to normal with accompanying pain for a week after the birth. When I called my wife this time (five and a half hours after birth), I was totally shocked to hear an alert, cheery voice answer the phone and tell me she had just finished a big breakfast and was going to take a shower. About twelve hours after birth she was ready to come home; it was only to abide by hospital rules that she stayed an additional forty hours in the hospital.

My only regret throughout the whole experience was that I forgot my camera on the dining-room table. Husbands, please note: Put your camera in your wife's suitcase so you don't forget it; and there's enough light in the delivery room to take color pictures. That is, of course, if your hospital and doctor allow you to take photographs.

Sincerely,

Jordan P.

Thomas

....

DEAR MRS. BING:

It was Saturday afternoon and the first time I had felt the heavy exhaustion of late pregnancy. I would rest tomorrow. I said to my husband, "I must be crazy, I know I still have two weeks to get ready for the baby, but I just had to do everything today."

A hot bath and early bed would make everything fine. It was 10 P.M. as I got out of the tub (my doctor does not restrict tub baths). There was a gush of water.

"My water has broken . . . the baby is coming . . . no, it's too soon! No," I recalled, "my doctor is out of town." I was scared; more than scared, I panicked. Perhaps if I would just go to bed, nothing would happen. My husband agreed, though we decided to warn my neighbor that our daughter, aged four, might have to be dropped off in the middle of the night. The neighbor convinced me that I should at least call the doctor who was substituting for mine. I was sure I could hold off until my own doctor got back into town—it would only be another eighteen hours. But I called anyhow, trying to sound very casual and unconcerned. My doctor's substitute said, "Come right in." I, doubtfully: "Are you sure? There are no contractions, and I do need some sleep!" But he insisted.

No! No! No! All my reading, my exercises, my classes did no good. I was convinced things were going to happen just like in my first delivery. I was tired, my doctor was not available, and now I had to go to the hospital too soon. The only difference was that last time I was naïvely unafraid and excited. Now I was frightened.

Did we dare call Mrs. Bing? We called, and she didn't mind. She agreed we should call the doctor once more and ask whether I could not get a little sleep before contractions started. She also said she was sure I would do fine, and she told my husband to be sure to come to what would have been our last class on Tuesday and tell all the other couples about our labor and delivery. This was the first ray of hope. How could she feel so certain everything would be a nice story on Tuesday? She must believe I could do it.

On the second call the doctor still insisted we get to the hospital immediately. I stalled about getting ready. We woke our little one and I told her, "We are going to the hospital. Maybe the baby is coming." She is so sweet, so wonderful. Yes, she was worth thirty-two miserable, lonely, confused hours of labor. She was worth the months of pain and exhaustion that crippled our beginnings of getting to know each other. But did it have to be like that again?

As we drove the twenty-mile trip to the hospital, mild contractions began. They were four, five, sometimes seven minutes apart. Actually they stayed just like that, except for their intensity, until I was in the delivery room.

The admitting clerk had been expecting us and was concerned. It was 1 A.M. I was admitted, and in the labor room a resident doctor examined me. It hurt, and there was no dilation and the uterus was not contracting very

123

much. My husband came to say good night and go to a hotel. The look of confusion on his face must have matched my own. Now I was alone.

With two sleeping pills, I slept about two hours. When I awoke, I started the slow, deliberate breathing exercises. Then I was told that my husband had come back. Thank heavens—I was afraid he would sleep through it all, and I wasn't there to wake him up. It was so good to see him; I devoured the lollipops he brought. The contractions were quite strong now, but I could get by with using the slow breathing. The doctor arrived and examined me. It was 8:30 A.M. I was 2 or 3 cm dilated. This was discouraging—almost 8 hours for so little dilation. He gave me pitocin, in the form of little flat pills to be put under the lip, to speed things up. I switched to the panting breathing, perhaps a little late, for I had trouble with it and soon switched to the transition breathing. This was fine, but I was sorry to have started so soon. I couldn't find a comfortable position except by walking around, which was against hospital rules. Finally I settled in the side position, with my husband massaging my abdomen. The contractions were very strong and moving into my back. The doctor returned again. It was 11:45 A.M. The dilation was 6 cm. I had hoped for more and said so, and I also said, "I am not going to make it. We have hours to go yet. Just like the first time. I can't make it!"

A contraction came. I tried to pant and lost it. I tensed against the pain and closed my eyes. It was excruciating. My husband said firmly, "Don't close your eyes. Look at me. Breathe!" And I followed his instructions. "It must have been a little one," I said. "No," he insisted, "it wasn't. Now look at me and follow my commands." Then I knew my fears would not overwhelm me; I trusted him and my confidence returned. About two contractions later I felt tremendous back pressure. Could it be the urge to push? I thought so. As soon as I said so, I was sure I was wrong. The doctor returned, examined me and said, "You can push now." He sent my husband to put on his delivery-room garb, and I was taken to the delivery room. Could it be true? Was it really time?

I was happy, tired and very anxious for my husband to get back. From then on I felt disconnected from my body. My thoughts were calm and controlled. My body seemed to be free-wheeling, doing what it had to do, quite independent of my will.

The anesthesiologist kept trying to hold the mask over my face, which was annoying, for then I held my breath when I should have been breathing. I wanted to slap it away but didn't dare, for I had promised not to move my hands if they would not strap me. The doctor was encouraging me to push. I was hesitant, for I recalled the stitches and hemorrhoids that had hurt me until my daughter was eighteen months old. On the third push, however, I gave way to my urge to push and pushed for all I was worth.

Everyone was giving orders. The doctor said, "Push," the anesthesiologist said, "Breathe, breathe deeply," my husband called out, "You're doing fine—push!" The nurse stood ready to strap my hands, in case I moved them. I needed time to collect myself and figure out whom to listen to and to practice what I had been taught. But there was no time, and I seemed to be able to push and breathe quite well spontaneously. I realized that the sensation going up my spine could have been pain, but I felt no pain. I felt the baby slipping out. The doctor said, "It's a gi—" I started to correct him before he corrected

125

himself. I knew it was a boy. Since I had started to push I had somehow known the baby well. He was placed on my stomach, and I heard myself saying over and over, "He looks just fine, he looks just fine!" It was 12:30 P.M.

As soon as the doctor had finished repairing the episiotomy, I did the pelvic floor exercises. I was exhausted and my legs ached from being in stirrups, but I lay there with a blissful smile on my face, listening to my baby cry.

This had not been childbirth "without fear." I was very afraid because of my memories from my first labor and delivery. But this time I had tools to fight the fear, and it seemed as if I now knew the miracle of being a woman.

Sincerely,
TERRY O.

A REPORT FROM THOMAS'S FATHER

DEAR MRS. BING:

You have asked me for a report about an experience that even the ablest writer would be at a loss to record. Words or pictures could only begin to describe the surface.

Having our first child was thirty hours of torture and, after we brought our baby girl home, a long period of mental depression for my wife, Terry. Neither of us was too eager for another child. When finally we did want a second, it was difficult to conceive for no apparent reason. Treatment by a specialist did result in success. With the promise of being a mother once again, Terry did not want to repeat her first experience. Through friends we found out about your classes and enrolled; and this time

126

the rewards were abundant. Being a very proud father of a new baby boy is only one of them.

From the beginning, it seemed that everything was going wrong. Terry lost her water first, with no contractions. Our doctor was out of town, and the attending physician insisted we come to the hospital. With much dragging of heels we went. Still no contractions. Again the hospital consumed Terry, and again I was at a loss, certain that we would never have the opportunity to use all we had been taught. However, by the next morning things started to happen, but not according to schedule. The contractions came at two-and-a-half-minute intervals for hours.

This time I was allowed to be with my wife. This time, rather than sitting alone waiting, thinking the worst about doctors, hospitals and medicine in general, I was actually allowed to enter the "secret place." The whole picture changed. What was it that I was supposed to do? My attitude changed too. This was no longer a chamber of horrors. The nurses and the whole staff were concerned and very efficient. A tremendous respect replaced my former contempt. We cannot applaud enough the attitudes and services of the hospital and our doctor who encouraged us to use the Lamaze method. I only hope more doctors will realize the gain of respect and trust that this can give the medical profession.

Slowly I remembered what I was supposed to be doing, what we had been taught. Terry was well in control, 3 centimeters dilated, and I timed her and massaged her back and abdomen for the next two or three hours.

Labor was progressing more rapidly. It looked as if it was getting painful. Terry looked weary. I thought, if it gets much worse, thumbs down on the whole thing and the doctor can knock her out. After four or five very strong contractions, Terry couldn't keep her eyes open. We were, I was sure, about to lose control. There is where I had to make my choice: to force her attention and work via me, or to let her progressively lose control and finally be medicated.

It worked—that is, I made my choice and forced her to work with me. By God, it worked. And then, after about five more strong contractions, the doctor examined her and said, "Go ahead, push!" The nurse started to get Terry ready for the delivery room. I was told where to change clothes, and I was in the delivery room at 12 noon. Even though I had met the doctor before, and of course seen him when he examined her each time in the labor room, I was very much relieved to see him right here in the delivery room. I felt like a second thumb, sure to get in the way, and I would have left willingly if the doctor had so much as pointed a finger at the door. Total respect for the man in charge replaced fear and doubt. Terry was afraid of having an episiotomy performed and voiced that fear. I, feeling that this was not the time for argument, reassured her that it was the doctor's decision and I was sure he would not perform one unless he had to.

It was 12:15 P.M. With each contraction the doctor directed, Terry pushed, and we all encouraged her. Terry seemed to push now with real purpose. I supported her back, watched her, tried to help her relax between contractions, and I saw my son born. It was 12:30 P.M. It seemed that everything inside me had slipped down to knee level. When I first came into this room I felt out of place. And now there could not have been any other place for me. I think the only person that felt unneeded was the anesthesiologist, though I was glad she was there, just in case. The doctor had performed an episiotomy, but Terry was all smiles, just looking at her baby boy—and we kissed.

I left to change into my street clothes again and went to have a cup of coffee. I met the doctor in the hall, and the only words I could get out were merely, "Thank you, Doctor." I had never understood how anyone could cry when they were happy, but now I was close to it.

When I saw my wife again she said, "All three of us have been born." She was right, and I was very proud of my wife, my son and myself.

Every woman should be encouraged to train for child-birth, every couple should train together. There is more to gain than just conquest of fears, a controlled delivery and a birth. There is an intense emotion that is beyond anything people can usually experience in a lifetime. There are many stories written about love, movies show us love, and we go through many fantasies in which a man and a woman are trying to find just this. When a man makes love to his wife, he wants her to achieve emotion uncontrolled, pleasure, pain, elation. This can happen when you are with her when she is giving birth to her child, and the exchange of love is indescribable. Then a man would never have to feel inadequate at lovemaking; a woman would never have to feel she was not a woman or mother. If she is conscious when she gives birth to her child, every part of her is a woman.

I must admit when I first agreed to go to the classes, I felt out of place. This was a woman's business, though something made me admit I had something to do with it. Up until the last half hour I seemed to be walking in a taboo area—and now—I laugh at it all and pity the man who fears it.

Sincerely,
ROBERT O.

Diane

DEAR MRS. BING:

I am sorry this report is a little late, but as you can well imagine, I have been pretty busy. I also hope that you won't find it to be too rambling, but I didn't want to leave anything out. I don't think I'll ever get over the thrill of seeing my daughter come into this world, and both my husband and I would be willing to go through the entire labor and delivery again tomorrow!

My due date was on Saturday, March 8th, and quite honestly we were convinced that I would give birth at any time, but not on my due date.

I awoke Saturday morning with a funny feeling in my abdomen, but really thought that I was imagining things. Not taking any chances, however, I immediately set my hair and went about last-minute cleaning chores in the house. I felt whatever it was about once every hour, and whatever it was lasted for thirty seconds. When my husband woke, I told him about this and we both decided to ignore these little signs and go about our business as usual.

We went out in the afternoon and didn't return until about 8 P.M., at which time we ate dinner. I ate lightly, to be on the safe side. I still only felt slight cramps every

130

hour, but they had gotten a little stronger. We were still convinced that all this was meaningless and by 12:30 A.M. went to sleep. Much to my surprise I found myself waking up every half hour with cramps that seemed a little sharper.

At 3 A.M. I woke my husband, and contractions were now coming every twenty minutes. He called the doctor and we were advised to come to the hospital. We dressed and were ready to go when the inevitable happened— contractions stopped coming. We waited a little while, and still nothing, but decided to get going anyway. We were both relieved when I felt something as we approached Triborough Bridge, as neither of us wanted to be told to go home once we had reached the hospital. I really wasn't sure whether I was in labor, as my membranes had not broken and I never had a bloody show, and I had no idea whether I was dilating or not.

However, once in the labor room, when I was examined by a resident, I was very happy to hear that I was already 4 cm dilated. I had used the first breathing technique then only when I felt I needed it. I was prepped and given an enema, and I found that contractions became more frequent and sharper while I was in the bathroom. I began the second breathing, panting in a 4-4 rhythm, combined with the first breathing exercise, as some of the contractions were not as strong as others.

When I returned to my room, the nurse called my husband. I didn't realize that one and a half hours had passed since our arrival, and my husband confided that when the nurse came to get him, he thought that she was going to tell him that I'd given birth by now.

My husband joined me by 5:30 A.M. and I gave him a progress report. He powdered my abdomen while I rubbed it, and we made quite a team. I had reached the lollipop stage and was really thankful that I had brought them. The nurse came in every ten minutes or so to listen to the fetal heart. She also put her hand on my stomach and told me when a contraction was coming, even before I felt it. Some of the contractions didn't last and were not as strong as others, and again I adjusted my breathing to what I felt at the time. Between contractions my husband and I joked and were taking bets as to what time of day we would be parents, and we finally decided that the baby would arrive by noon.

By 6:30 A.M. the contractions came at six- to seven-minute intervals and lasted from forty to sixty seconds. I was using the panting in a 4-4 rhythm, and my husband kept on putting powder on my belly and wetting the washcloth for me. Bringing the washcloth was also a very good idea as it was very refreshing to be able to suck a few drops of water.

At 7:15 A.M. my doctor came to examine me and found I was 6 cm dilated. He told us that we would probably have the baby by 10:30 A.M. Soon afterward, the contractions increased in strength considerably. Up to that time I had been sitting on the edge of the bed with feet dangling or I had rested on the bed with my back well supported and my knees raised. Nobody came in to tell me that I had to sit or lie in any particular position.

By 8 A.M. the contractions were coming at three-minute intervals and lasting sixty to ninety seconds. I began to use the third breathing technique combined with the second. The point came where I didn't feel there was any relief between contractions. The nurse popped her head in and asked if I wanted a sedative. I said no, but two seconds later I asked my husband to get the doctor and said that I needed some help. The doctor came in and found that I could start with pushing, and I forgot about the medication. By 8:30 A.M. I was wheeled into the delivery room. I was so glad they did not take my glasses away from me and that nobody tied my wrists down. I kept pushing with each contraction and my husband helped by giving my shoulders support. At 8:45 A.M., with a final push, I saw my daughter's head emerge. As far as I was concerned this was the most beautiful sight in the world! As soon as the head was out I felt wonderful. She was already crying, and as soon as the doctor had her whole body out, she began to cry frantically, without any further stimulation. Soon after, the doctor pushed on my abdomen and the placenta came out. I had been ready to push it out myself, but he told me to relax, which I did.

Then they brought me my baby, and to my eyes she was the most beautiful baby in the world. My husband was allowed to hold her also in the delivery room. The doctor explained to my husband that he was now repairing the episiotomy and that I was getting a fancy Sunday special stitch.

I really felt wonderful and couldn't understand (and still can't) how some women act half dead for many days after delivery.

As far as my husband and I are concerned, the birth of our daughter was the greatest experience of our lives. Without the help of my husband, I doubt whether I could have made it. He gave me moral support and was a tremendous help in making me physically comfortable. We were both gratified that the nurse did not stay in the room all the time; I do not think that I would have felt very relaxed with a stranger present all the time. As it was, we felt free to talk about whatever we wished, and we also knew that if help was needed, the nurses were just a few steps away.

I can honestly say that I do not feel that *I* gave birth to our baby, but rather that *we* gave birth.

And here is a little criticism of myself: when the contractions began to come hard and fast, I panicked occasionally, and was not as relaxed as I should have been. Now that I know what to expect, I hope to do better next time!

It really seems strange to me that I know more about pregnancy and labor and delivery than some women who have had two or more children, who seem to have not the slightest idea of what happened to them during their nine months of carrying their baby, and who seem to have even less knowledge about labor and delivery. Knowing what to expect and how to work along with it, rather than fearing the unknown, is indeed knowledge worth while acquiring. We are both so happy that we took the time to find out what pregnancy, labor and delivery are all about.

Yours,
GAIL J.

Sean Patrick

DEAR MRS. BING:

It's very difficult to begin this report to you and contain my enthusiasm for the Lamaze method and for your instructions.

Labor for me was quick (perhaps one and one-half hours of uncertainty as to whether I was actually in labor or not) and almost immediately involved long and hard contractions.

At 1:30 A.M. I awakened my husband—who then set about dressing himself, getting things generally organized, all between my contractions, which he was timing with a stopwatch. Once he was up, it seemed the contractions became progressively harder, which, as I reflect on it now, must have meant I woke him at the best moment.

I had *all* the symptoms: vomiting and shaking. When we finally called my doctor, he felt that since this was my first baby, I was in the early phases of labor, which, of course, had been my idea too, except I didn't feel I could stand it for any fifteen hours, and I told him so over the phone. As a contraction began I asked him to hold on till I was finished and my husband held the phone and counted out the time to me from the stopwatch. As he reached and passed seventy-five seconds, the doctor interrupted and said he would meet us at the hospital.

We took our time and finally got down to our car. The bucket seats of the car made this part of labor the easiest. I was also going through periods of being very warm and opening the windows and very cold and closing them and enjoying the heat in the car.

I was at this time combining every tool at my disposal: shallow breathing, panting and blowing—using them together. I had actually done this most of the time at home, much to my dismay, since I now remembered your telling us not to use everything straight away.

My husband asked me while we were on our way if he should drive fast or slow, and I told him slow, since we would probably wind up staring at one another for another fifteen hours.

At the hospital doorway (and it was raining), I had a strong contraction and totally ignored the rain and the attendant offering me a chair. My husband told him I was "just having a contraction and will be all right in a minute."

We finally got upstairs. My husband left to fill out the papers and get something to eat and the nurse set about trying to get me into a gown between contractions (when I was in one, per your instructions I totally ignored everybody around me) and into bed. Immediately I asked for the bed to be raised and was told that my doctor had to examine me first. He did and said I would have the baby soon, and I asked how long soon was.

Very soon I was taken into another room, which for lack of a term I've been titling the "expulsion room." A little Irish student nurse at this point was the most invaluable person to me and one I will always remember. She told me I could push, and I insisted on seeing my doctor—I thought it was too soon to push and that she was telling

136

me the wrong thing. She convinced me, but I was starting to fall apart, until she asked if I'd had instructions. I said yes, and she said to me, "Surely you know what position to take up for pushing?" and she helped me up. When I pushed I strained my neck instead of using my abdominal muscles, and she noticed it and corrected me. And then I remembered and everything came back to me, and I proceeded to do what I had been taught because there was nothing else to do but just that.

Next came the delivery room—they asked me to get on the table, which I was not at all ready to do, and I would have just stayed on the bed and had the baby there. I asked my husband if he would help me, and he moved my bottom while the nurse, in vain, tried to move my shoulders—and so my husband moved me entirely onto the table. He was wonderfully helpful.

The rest followed like a classroom lesson. Then the baby was born. I practically jumped right off the table and the doctor asked me to lean back, as it looked as if I might fall off the table.

Then came the time to expel the placenta, and I asked to do it myself, and boom, boom, it was all over and I can't recollect any discomfort—in fact my husband reminded me tonight that I did it all by myself, the expulsion of the placenta, and not the doctor, and I'd already forgotten. And yet, my sister, for example, remembers the expulsion of the placenta as a miserable experience.

Having seen our baby being born will always be one of the great memories in our lives—in fact, I can't even conjure up a moment that has occurred or might occur in the future that could compare in any way to our experience in giving birth to our baby. To think that so very many girls and women have not had a similar experience, or that their husbands could not share it with them, saddens me. That such a beautiful experience in life should be missed for foolish reasons such as pure ignorance, i.e., lack of education, seems a great shame. I felt so secure knowing what to expect and how to cope with contractions. And, above all, there was the emotional satisfaction I experienced. This was my first baby and my pregnancy was wonderful, I had no fears, nor was I apprehensive once I had learned how to cope with my labor and delivery.

I've never been able to stand any sort of pain . . . in fact, I got into a cold sweat when I thought of a needle. But you gave me "tools," and even though I still had uncomfortable moments, I could work with my contractions and also was still able to choose drugs if I felt I needed them.

When the placenta came out, I said to the doctor, "Don't throw it away." And later he gave my husband and me a lesson on the placenta and we were fascinated.

Now I can't imagine having the baby any other way. Nor can I fathom how a woman can give birth in ignorance. If I hadn't known what to do, I don't think I would ever have the courage to have another baby. It would have been too painful and traumatic an experience.

After the birth of our baby, and while the doctor was patching me up, the doctor, my husband and I had a smashing time. We joked, discussed all kinds of things, and my husband after a while went to get some coffee, which we shared together when I was back in my room.

Well—I've heard how brave I am; how great I am; how well I did, though others probably couldn't do it. My reaction is just to keep silent. I can't really tell and explain that this was the greatest moment in our marriage. I came to you to learn because I was scared and needed help.

138

I'll be seeing you hopefully in about fifteen months for a refresher class.

> Sincerely.
> JACQUELINE F.

Jonathan

••

DEAR MRS. BING:

Before I tell you about my wonderful experience, I'd just like to tell you about my frustrating time prior to giving birth. As you know, my due date was originally estimated for April 5th. But that was a great miscalculation. I didn't have the baby until May 14th. And between neighbors and anxious grandparents-to-be, not to mention how my husband and I felt, I really suggest that all future mothers tell everyone that the due date is at least two weeks later than the given time. And if it comes early, then it's just a lovely surprise for all.

Well, now that that is off my chest, down to my big day of days. At 3:45 Tuesday morning my waters broke, though I didn't realize at first that that was what was happening. I just felt that I had to go to the bathroom, which was not unusual. On my way back to bed, water was running down my legs. So back to the bathroom. This happened twice. The second time it happened I noticed some blood with it, and the flow was longer, and then I knew what it was. I called my husband quietly, because I was so excited and had to share my wonderful news. He was very pleased and we stood there giggling at each other. And then we went back to bed, as nothing else had hap-

140

pened. At 5 A.M. I started to get some very mild contractions which were six minutes apart. I kept checking with my stopwatch and I was surprised that they came so frequently right away. I decided not to wake my husband again and tried to get some sleep myself. But by 6 A.M. I woke my husband. He was very calm and we decided to call the doctor at 6:30 A.M. He told me to take my time, get dressed slowly and come to the hospital by 9 A.M. I really couldn't believe I was finally going to have my baby.

At the hospital I was taken to a labor room, and after I had been prepped, my husband joined me, and as contractions were still fairly easy, we decided to play cards. When the doctor examined me, he said that I was doing fine, but that he wanted to speed up the contractions, as they were not strong enough. This was done intravenously. The contractions got stronger. My husband was great—he helped me by cooling my face, keeping time and watching over me all the time. I still used the first breathing technique, and I found the massaging helped me to relax well. I was most comfortable sitting up, though not sitting up absolutely straight.

The contractions got harder and I had to use the second breathing pattern. I really had to concentrate hard, and my husband found a spot for me to concentrate on. It was a little light over the doorway, and on a piece of white tape that he stuck to it, he wrote, "I love you." And that helped me a great deal.

At about 2 P.M. the doctor examined me again and I was only 3 cm dilated. I received some Demerol to help me relax. I was getting tired and needed every bit of rest between contractions. They were coming now one and a half to two minutes apart, and I was not even halfway dilated. All this time my husband reminded me to relax, which helped a great deal. By 5 p.m. my doctor examined me again and found I had progressed to 5 cm. Things were looking up a bit, but he felt it would still take quite a while. The second breathing technique didn't help at this point. I would start panting, then, as the contraction got harder, it would take my breath away, and I could manage then by blowing only. My husband would do the blowing with me and I was able to follow him. My poor husband never got any dinner—he had to work so hard with me.

The doctor examined me again and I was 8 cm dilated. He said it would take about twenty more minutes, and I could start pushing. This seemed to be the most beautiful news I had heard in a long time. And strangely enough I couldn't really believe it. But soon the doctor said, "Let's go," and he handed my husband white pants and shirt, and down the hall we went, and I still couldn't believe it.

I was wheeled into the delivery room, and the next thing that happened was that they told me to get onto the table. I felt they might have helped me a bit. Ah, well, I got on. My husband remembered to put pillows under my head, and everything was very exciting now. I was tired and so busy that I can't quite remember all the details. My husband says the student nurses were really excited now. The doctor told me to push with my next contraction, but strangely enough I could not tell when it began. Again my husband helped and told me when, because he saw my belly harden. He said it looked so funny. I pushed and pushed, and then the resident helped by pushing down on my abdomen, and my husband urged, "Push, push, push," and I did. I could feel the baby's head trying to get out, and I was trying to see it in the

142

mirror, but it was not in the exact position for me to see and everyone was too busy to adjust it. So I picked my head up further and I watched my beautiful child being born. The first thing he did was to sneeze, and then he cried. The doctor said, "It's a boy," and I called out his name, "Jonathan!"

You see, Mrs. Bing, it was quite difficult and long, but I'd do it again. The best thing was my husband praising me after a really hard contraction.

By now Jonathan weighs 11.2 pounds and is twenty-four inches long, and we are a very happy family.

Sincerely,
DIANE L.

Dana Michelle

DEAR MRS. BING:

At about 11:30 A.M. on Friday, February 7, I received a message while in court that my wife would appreciate a call from me. Realizing that Sukey had been in the first phases of labor for better than twenty-four hours, it wasn't difficult for me to conclude that this time she wasn't calling me to ask me to pick something up at the store.

I called her and she informed me that the doctor had called her and advised her to come to the hospital. She said she had not yet commenced first-stage breathing nor were the contractions coming at fairly regular or sustained intervals.

I arrived home about 12 noon and since Sukey didn't appear to be in any pain or difficulty, I proceeded to have lunch and read the mail.

At about 12:30 P.M. we left for the hospital, but not before I had Sukey pose for a few photographs in her pregnant state. On the way to the hospital we dropped our dog off at my parents' house and my mother could not get over how casual and relaxed we both were about the whole thing.

Actually we felt that it was a bit early to be going to

the hospital, but we decided that before we checked in with the admissions office we would have the doctor check Sukey to make sure this was the real thing.

On the way to the hospital, both of us were very relaxed and I was very confident that we could handle the situation with a minimum of discomfort. We had been practicing regularly, though for the past two weeks we had stopped the relaxation exercises.

Sukey was examined by the doctor and I was then informed that we would be staying, since Sukey was about 1 cm dilated and the doctor had punctured the membranes. I tried to convince them that with such a small dilation we could be here for hours and it would be psychologically tiring to Sukey, but it was to no avail; they told me to check her in.

After what appeared to be an inordinate length of time, Sukey was brought to the labor room at about 2:15 P.M. She looked fine and was smiling, and I could tell she had just gone through an interesting experience. She had heard that the worst part of delivery was the prepping and enema. "Well," she said, "if the enema is supposed to be the worst part of this thing, I should do OK."

Sukey was half sitting, and as the contractions came and went she would use the first-level breathing only for the severe portion of the contraction. At this point her breathing and concentration were excellent and her ability to relax was good.

My role during this first period was minimal. I watched her relaxation, and she also desired firm rubbing pressure along both sides of the abdomen. At times it was difficult to determine exactly where she wanted me to rub, but she was usually able to guide my hands to the proper place.

Sukey began the second breathing about 3 P.M. Her

breathing and concentration were good, but she was not sufficiently relaxing during the contractions. She recognized this inability to relax completely, and though I urged her to "relax—relax," it did not always help.

At 3:45 P.M. a nurse checked Sukey and informed her she was about 3 cm dilated. The contractions were still coming irregularly, between six and three minutes, and lasted about twenty to thirty seconds. By 4 P.M Sukey asked me to exert great pressure on her thigh. She was still in complete control, but her ability to relax was diminishing.

By 4:45 P.M. my notes say, Sukey was "very worm." I really don't think I was feeling that she was a worm, but she was beginning to show the first signs of irritability. The contractions were also getting notably stronger. By 5:10 P.M. I told her to change to transition breathing.

As soon as she went to the pant-blow breathing, she was able to regain control. I also breathed along with her more frequently than I had done before. I think Sukey merely enjoyed my blowing into her face, and it is doubtful whether my breathing actually helped her in hers.

At 5:30 P.M. two nurses came in at my request to check dilation. I was informed that Sukey was 7 cm dilated and that she should deliver by 7 P.M. The nurse called the sixth floor and told them that "She'll be down by seven o'clock. Have her dinner ready!" I proceeded to dance up and down the hall!

At about 6:30 P.M. Sukey began to lose control of her contractions. When I would try and get her to pant-blow, both by doing it and suggesting it, she would tell me that she was doing what felt best. I should have been much firmer with her at this point. My notes say that by 6:45 P.M. Sukey was "not friendly." Clearly she was getting very tired and was still very warm.

146

At 7:42 p.m. the doctor came in and made an internal check, and the result was rather disappointing. He told us that the contractions were not strong enough and it might take another two hours. However, he also said that if we wanted the baby by about 8:30 p.m. he could arrange it! Sukey was given an intravenous solution of water, glucose and pitocin. The placing of the needle was not entirely painless and I recall the doctor saying something like "Sukey's elephant skin."

The doctor had brought another nurse with him, and she immediately grasped the situation and took over. Sukey was told to relax—she did. Sukey was told to concentrate—she did. Sukey was told to pant-blow—she did. The nurse told her, "You can do it," and gave her confidence and encouragement.

At about 8:20 p.m. the doctor told Sukey she could push. And did she push! She was able to hold her breath for at least forty-five seconds on each first push and for about thirty to thirty-five seconds on the second push. She was doing marvelously and we were all having fun shouting encouragements to her. I was talking to her constantly: "Come on, Sukey, push, push, push harder, Suke. Keep pushing; you can hold on, now really push, that's it! Now hold on for just ten more seconds, one, two, three. . . ."

After the second push, the doctor said he could see a dime's worth of the baby's head. He told me to watch during the next contraction. It was the most exciting event in my life! When I saw it, I think I said something like this: "There it is, Suke! There it is! I can see it moving. It's beautiful! Keep pushing. Push, push. It's beautiful, it's beautiful!"

Then at about 8:30 p.m. she was taken into the delivery room and was still in complete control of her contractions. At about 8:49 p.m. Suke gave one good push and out the baby came. The doctor was holding the baby by its feet and I said, "There he is, Suke, there he is." The doctor corrected me and said, "No, it's not a he, it's a girl." And so Dana Michelle was born, and all parties were in perfect physical and mental condition. We were quietly ecstatic.

Suggestions to Future Lamaze Husbands:

1. Practice relaxation and breathing exercises every day. I had mastered the breathing; I would check myself occasionally.

2. Be firm and loving and talk Lamaze. The nurse at the end showed me that Sukey had everything she needed for a perfect Lamaze delivery. But I had not been sufficiently firm with her; I did not force her to try the pant-blow breathing, for instance. As a husband, you should expect a certain level of performance from your wife. You should be confident prior to labor that she can reach this level of performance and then you should see that she does in fact perform.

It was a totally beautiful experience. I eagerly await our next child, for I believe we can be nearly perfect Lamaze students, and the experience of birth is much too exhilarating to have happen only once in a lifetime!

Sincerely,

GILBERT G.

Khela Dawn

DEAR MRS. BING:

March 3rd came and went without the birth of our child. Monday, the fourth, bright and early, I departed on my usual city excursions consisting of exploring new spots in Mayor Lindsay's fun city. I could not possibly bear to stay at home and answer the many calls that were bound to come from curious friends and relatives. The day went very smoothly and I arrived home at 5 P.M.; just in time for the first signs of my preliminary labor. (The contractions were very mild and came every twenty to thirty minutes, lasting about fifteen seconds.) My husband called from work asking if I'd like to meet him in the city to take in a show. Never passing up an opportunity to go out, I left for the city once again, minutes after his call. We grabbed a bite to eat (pizza), which I suppose I should have passed up, but I decided one slice couldn't hurt.

At around 6:30 P.M. we entered the movies. Ironical as it may seem, we saw *The Whisperers*. So at the beginning of a new life we sat watching a film about the problems of old age and loneliness.

Now the contractions were coming every ten to fifteen minutes, lasting twenty seconds. Unfortunately we forgot to bring a watch. Near the end of the movies I felt the need to do the deep breathing exercises, which were very helpful. We left the movies around 8 P.M. and walked leisurely to the subway, stopping to do the exercises as the need arose. We stopped in a bookstore, browsed around and bought a book.

The contractions were now coming every eight to ten minutes, lasting thirty seconds, approximately, and we decided to head for home. I felt that in addition to the exercises, I needed the security of holding onto my husband with one hand, thus leaving only one to rub my tummy.

The journey on the subway was more difficult than my earlier experiences. The contractions were coming about every five minutes and, although lasting about thirty seconds, were much stronger than previously. I definitely needed to do the exercises, and at first I was somewhat embarrassed to do so because of the many people around. But need overcame modesty and feelings of self-consciousness, and I soon blocked out all but the breathing techniques and my husband.

Finally at 9:30 P.M. we arrived home, and what a good feeling it was. Now we were ready to really buckle down to business. The contractions were coming every five minutes and lasting forty-five seconds. We worked very hard together. I suppose I was well conditioned, because I would automatically begin the breathing with each contraction. However, I needed my husband to remind me not to become sloppy and forget the cleansing breaths and occasionally rubbing the tummy.

Since I was so certain I was going to be late and had much time before the birth of the baby, I hadn't packed my suitcase or little bag for the labor room. So in between contractions we hustled around making peanut butter and jelly sandwiches (which nearly turned my stomach) and packed tangerines. All this food was for my husband. We got powder, washcloth and lollipops together and loaded my husband's pockets.

At about 10:15 P.M. the contractions were coming every three minutes and the labor was shifting from abdominal to low back discomfort. I now switched to the panting since it seemed more helpful. You were right, I did the panting with much more ease and even rhythm now in labor than I was able to do in class. We decided to call the doctor and let him know of my progress. He suggested we come to the hospital. I was sure it was too early, I was not very uncomfortable, even though the contractions were coming three minutes apart, and I did not want to be sent home again. However, the low back pain was exerting pressure on my rectum and I thought perhaps I should be examined anyway. So at 10:30 we departed.

At this point I would like to interject that my husband was marvelous and so very calm. So calm that on the way to the hospital he would stop the car with each of my contractions to time them. Finally I had to tell him it wasn't really necessary to stop with each contraction.

At 11 P.M. we arrived at the hospital. Of all things, they want you to fill out papers and sign others. Just what I felt like doing! I finally made the labor room, coming in contact with many unhelpful people on the way. I met the nurse, who insisted I stop trembling and that I put my knees down during the peak of a contraction so that she could listen to the fetal heart.

Finally the resident came in to examine me and he refused to utter any information other than "Your baby will be here soon."

I now had a strong urge to push and I was panting and attempting to blow with the urge to push. At long last my husband was allowed to come into the labor room. I can't possibly express what a great comfort it was to have him there. I felt such a deep love for this man who was soon to be a daddy.

I was able to find one understanding nurse who told me I was 7 cm dilated. However, the most overwhelming urge to push, which I was now experiencing, was the most difficult phase of my labor. Finally my doctor arrived, examined me and came in with some scopolamine and Demerol, which I refused to take. I really felt like punching him. I didn't, of course, but I felt that things were difficult enough without having two people with conflicting philosophies attempting to work together.

Finally I was told I could push, and I did so with every ounce of strength in my body. Things were suddenly no longer difficult, although my husband was sure I was even more uncomfortable from the grunting sounds I was uttering. I was wheeled into the delivery room and within fifteen minutes Khela Dawn was leaving the warm confines of utero to begin her life.

It was a beautiful, moving experience for me. My only regrets are that my husband, who worked so hard with me, was not allowed to reap the reward of seeing his first little daughter enter this world.

Sincerely,
HELEN C.

Amanda

DEAR MRS. BING:

Here's something I bet you thought you'd never get—a report from us. I am sure you gathered from our phone call in December how ecstatic we were and are. And, of course, how busy. No more Christmas babies for us!

By the way, our daughter was named Amanda, and I put in an order for Amanda's little brother while still on the delivery table. So I hope before too long we'll be coming to class again. Perhaps I can learn my breathing better this time, or at least learn to slow down my switch from deep breathing to panting.

Both of us are extremely grateful for all the help and encouragement you gave us. With a pregnancy as good as mine was, and the actual labor and delivery well controlled through use of the Lamaze method, having babies is a true pleasure. We now wonder why we waited so long to start our family. My next baby will be born using the Lamaze method. I wouldn't think of going into another labor without the aids of the method to rely on.

My approach to the breathing was probably faulty, but from the beginning of labor my contractions were coming at completely regular intervals of three minutes, lasting forty to forty-five seconds. They never slowed or stopped, and they gradually increased in intensity. I had to walk about ten blocks to the hospital and I believe this hurried things along. For some reason I found the effleurage (massage of the abdomen), which had felt so comforting during my practice sessions to be distracting in actual labor and I was never able to use it. Instead I held my hands to the bottom of my abdomen as one would during transition.

Soon after I was prepped, deep breathing did not seem sufficient and I switched to panting. If I could have avoided this, I would have had a smoother labor. My husband, who was extremely helpful in timing my contractions, keeping my face wiped with a damp cloth and supplying me with crushed ice and courage, had no alternative suggestion to get me away from the early panting.

The resident doctor was a young Filipino woman, obviously witnessing her first birth by the Lamaze method. She refused to admit that I was in labor until I had been in the hospital about two hours; she continually urged me to take medication; she ruptured my membranes without telling me that she was going to do so or without telling me afterward what she had done (not that there was any doubt); and finally, when I was on the delivery table, she leaned over and said. "You aren't even going to let the doctor use forceps?" I found her whole attitude enraging, and I might add she seemed startled to see me up and about the next day as she was making her rounds in the maternity ward.

Because I had started my panting very early, I was exhausted when I reached the transition phase. The doctor said he thought that it would be another two or two and one-half hours till delivery. At this point he was giving me a great deal of encouragement, but I began to feel too tired to attempt to stay in control for two more hours. My contractions had become extremely irregular and I was getting no rest between. I asked for Demerol, but the doctor refused to give it to me. He said that I was so tired that Demerol would put me to sleep and I would not be awake for the delivery. After a very logical argument by him, I consented to a paracervical block.

I was wheeled directly into the delivery room. As soon as the block was administered I began to feel the contractions with much less intensity, but was told to push with each contraction. Sometimes, because of the block, I would not be sure when a contraction was building, and the doctor would put his hand on my abdomen to tell me when it was time to push. My husband, at the head of the delivery table, supported my back with each push. I began to feel in complete control and was just upset that it seemed to be taking so long. Now I realize that it seemed longer because I was doing pushing on the delivery table, a pushing which normally would have been done first in the labor room.

At the end I felt some pain when the baby began to press hard on the perineum, but I never lost control. From time to time the doctor would call my husband to the foot of the table to see what progress was being made. He told my husband that I was turning the baby's head by pushing so well.

The doctor made the episiotomy, and with the next push I could feel the baby's head, and its body being born —I could feel each part of the body. That's the first time I let out a yell, a yell of joy. It was a moment I will never forget. My husband was yelling too and the doctor was holding up our daughter, who sneezed immediately and then started to cry. As soon as the cord was cut, I pushed the placenta out.

I had been experiencing hunger pangs between contractions for quite some time, and my husband went off to get us some food. The hours of lying on the table for observation was dreadful and endless, but I guess this is the price you have to pay for being awake.

In my case, I feel that the paracervical block was the perfect answer because I would have been too tired to last and to participate in my daughter's birth otherwise.

I hope that with my next labor I will have better control over my breathing so that I won't have to ask for medication.

My doctor commended me again on my pushing when I went for my six-weeks' checkup. He said that I was the best Lamaze patient he had ever had, which I don't think means anything, because I don't think he's had that many, but at least he's willing to give me more support with the next baby, and he was convinced that my husband was an asset in the delivery room. He actually hates to have husbands in the delivery room, but he felt that mine, through his training, was a real asset.

Goodbye and thank you till the next time.

Sincerely,
ADELE L.

A Recapitulation
of the Training Session

EDITOR'S NOTE: The following item is not a report from a happy new father; it is an account of one of my lessons, which he attended. His wife took a daytime course, to which he could not accompany her regularly. However, I encourage my students to try and bring their husbands at least once to a session and thus hopefully get a fair idea of the hard task which their wives will have to face in the near future.

After four sessions of training in various breathing techniques, my wife invited me to accompany her to a more general session, or dress rehearsal, where other husbands were also to be present. Two of the husbands had attended all the sessions to date. On this particular Thursday there were about a dozen women, the two regular husbands, myself and four more men—some of the women had not been able to arrange for their husbands to come.

I found the two-hour session fascinating in two ways. For one thing, Mrs. Bing's gentle, informal chat about the whole process of labor and delivery recapitulated a great deal of practical information from the previous sessions and put the whole Lamaze method into a sensible perspective. Although I have two sons in their late teens, I had never before been involved in the process, and I learned a great deal that made good, practical sense.

But even more fascinating was the opportunity to observe the effect on a dozen prospective mothers of this sort of training. A few had had children before, most were to deliver their first. All of them seemed to be in their late twenties or early thirties (my wife, at thirty-five, was the oldest there). All seemed to be well above average intelligence and intellectual interest in approaching an age-old problem in a new way. All were good solid middle class —some conventional, some avant-garde.

Since I had been in town during the morning, I arrived early at an apartment block near the Museum of Natural History. A buzzer let me through the front door into a lobby with ugly tile floors and walls covered by many layers of paint. A very mixed bag of West Side denizens accompanied me in the elevator to the sixth floor.

Mrs. Bing's door was ajar, and I stuck my head in, very tentatively announcing that I was "Inge's husband." Mrs. Bing and the two or three women already there seemed to know who I was.

Mrs. Bing was seated at a small desk, chatting with the other women. I found one of the aluminum chairs and took a seat to listen. The chairs were all around the wall, facing the center of a large living room. Around the walls were some excellent photographs of various stages of labor, delivery, and the baby, including some of primitive sculptures —pre-Columbian art from Mexico.

Conversation was general. Mrs. Bing took time to talk to a prospective student about the choice of hospitals and obstetricians on the telephone, and chatted with the other women about her new air-conditioning unit in the window.

From time to time the buzzer would sound, and Mrs. Bing would walk the length of the room and push the signal that let another student through the entrance door below. The women drifted in, some with husbands and some without. Several went into the waiting room to leave street clothing, to change into slacks, or to go to the bathroom.

My own wife eventually arrived, kissed me nicely and went to leave her skirt in the waiting room, wearing dark tights for the exercises.

When all the women had arrived, Mrs. Bing started to go through the whole process from the onset of labor, going to the hospital, what to take, how to get what you want from the hospital staff, how labor progresses, the doctor's role, delivery, nursing and care of the baby in the hospital, and coming home. Sometimes she would question to bring out whether the students had learned their lessons. Sometimes she had them go through the breathing exercises and the pushing exercise. Sometimes she calmly provided new information in a highly organized but quite informal manner.

I listened carefully but watched the other people in the room. Everyone had their eyes on Mrs. Bing—partially because of genuine interest in what she was saying and partially to avoid looking at other people in the room. One of the regular husbands (who may have been a doctor himself) was either taking copious notes or drawing rude sketches of other people in the room.

Some of the women had learned their lessons and were very serious about giving answers to questions. They were subdued, in general, probably because of all these strange men in the group for the first time, during a frank dis-

159

cussion of some pretty intimate details. One did not do any of the exercises because her doctor had told her that she had started to dilate. That reminded another to tell Mrs. Bing that one woman would not be present at all that day, for the same reason. One or two didn't put much heart into the demonstration exercises. It could have been, "I'm lazy," or "Oh, I know all about that, I don't have to go through it again." It could have been, "I don't really want to with all these strangers here."

There was real love and openness among the women— a very strong sense of mutual dependence. Based on my own wife's reactions from week to week and her reports of what had happened, I am sure that there was a general thawing of one woman to all others. The accurate and continual use of correct medical terminology helped to make the whole future experience easier to talk about.

Mrs. Bing's frank appraisal of what a hospital staff would do and wouldn't do, her vivid description of the "hurricane hour" (transition), her explanation of when what would hurt and why, her methodical enumeration of wide variations from the norm, all helped to eliminate the mystery. Her calm manner instilled a sense of trust. Her anecdotes made it clear that she knew what she was talking about and her words could be accepted with complete faith.

As I said at the beginning, I learned a great deal about childbirth and about the Lamaze method that I expect to be of considerable practical help in about two weeks. But I was also impressed with the value of the six weeks of training as something in itself.

A woman who is pregnant for the first time knows that something quite different from any previous experience is going to happen. Old wives' tales (literally) can be very frightening. There is a great feeling of loneliness and of having tremendous responsibility to bear.

Just the process of meeting for two hours once a week with a dozen others in the same boat creates a healthy interdependence that goes a long way to eliminate the sense of loneliness—one or two of the couples seemed to be people it might be nice to know in later years.

The Lamaze breathing techniques undoubtedly do make it possible to cope with the pain effectively and to be an intelligent participant in the delivery. But beyond that, Mrs. Bing's own aura of competence and experience generated confidence in herself for each of the students. Not only was there a freedom from the fright of the unknown, and a freedom from the fear of intense pain, but also a freedom to believe in one's own capability and fulfillment.

I would have said that I hadn't much to do, no necessary role. I don't think that my wife—who has studied her lessons intensely—needs anyone to tell her when to breathe by what method. She's fully competent to do that herself. But somehow, out of the whole discussion, and the observation of the group as a whole (it wasn't a dozen and a half individuals, but a viable and effective group as a unit), I found a very necessary role for myself during labor and delivery. In some intangible but important way I'm part of the process, and it will be our baby because of my participation, not just my wife's baby.

The unifying and freeing experience of being a member of a group, and not a lonely, frightened woman, seems to me to be quite as important as the breathing techniques of the Lamaze method.

Shirley Jane

DEAR MRS. BING:

Here is the second part of our saga: The first part was my account of the training session which I attended. I then just jotted down my impressions of the lesson. The "second chapter" involved me so much more that I want to address the letter to you, personally.

On Wednesday, April 30th, my wife began to feel very uncomfortable and found it hard to lie in any position in which she could sleep. The original target date had been the day before, Tuesday, but on the Monday evening our obstetrician had said that we couldn't expect the baby until the weekend. Thursday she felt much better, and by Friday was in top spirits, feeling rested and relaxed, and ready to go on a trip to Europe.

Saturday morning I woke about 3 A.M. to find that she had gone to the kitchen to drink some milk and read while sitting up. The water had broken about midnight, flooding her with hot water, which she said was surprising. She had a few mild contractions, but came back to bed at 4 A.M. and slept soundly until 8:30.

Throughout the morning the contractions came at about seven-to-ten-minute intervals, and she had a chance to discover the value of controlled breathing to ease the discom-

162

fort. By 1:30 they were coming at four-minute intervals, some very strong, so we called the doctor and headed for the hospital, half an hour away.

Luckily we found a parking space right in front of the door, but walking about seemed to aggravate the contractions, and a very strong one arrived just as she went up the five steps. So she had to stop and try to get control before going on. When she could get some warning of when the next was due by watching the stopwatch, the breathing helped considerably. But when the contraction started strongly and took her by surprise, I had to do a fair amount of coaching to get her to breathe correctly, and those contractions could be quite painful.

After the pain subsided, she turned to go in and tripped over the bags I had set on the floor to help her. The scraped shinbone didn't seem to be a sufficient counter-irritant later on, however.

It was surprisingly easy to register at Mt. Sinai Hospital. In the admissions office the young man at the typewriter looked up and asked, "Mrs. Brown?" When I said yes, he said, "You wait in the waiting room while I take Mrs. Brown upstairs. You can go up in about half an hour." When he came back down I had only to show him my Blue Cross certificate and sign the financial responsibility statement. Somebody somewhere has worked out a system to get all the necessary details down onto all the necessary forms without flap. It sort of restores one's faith in organization.

A little before three the receptionist sent me up with the bags. My wife had had all her preparations, and was sitting in a chair having a contraction. The hospital was very quiet that afternoon, with only one other woman in labor. The nurses flitted in and out and were most helpful and understanding. One who spotted my wife's English accent said that she had trained for eight years in London, and apparently had had lots of experience with the Lamaze method.

I tried to help by coaxing my wife to relax during the contractions and to breathe regularly. One of the nurses explained the need for more oxygen during the contractions. The contractions progressed regularly, becoming very much stronger. By about five the pain really became unbearable (this was her first child) and no amount of coaching could keep her relaxed and breathing under control during the contraction. Between times she did manage to relax very well and get some rest. But the obstetrician decided that she would have to have medication to relieve the pain. So at 5:30 she became sleepy, and I was sent down to the waiting room.

I read John Gunther's *Twelve Cities*. About 6:30 the doctor came down and said that he expected it would take about another thirty minutes. At 7:30, when I had gotten halfway into Moscow, he came down again, and said that a baby girl was born at 7:09 and that everybody was fine. I could see them in about ten minutes.

The waiting room was quite full just then for the start of evening visiting hours, and several people smiled at us in the nicest way.

I went up to the nursery to see Shirley Jane, weighing seven pounds four ounces, being given a thorough bath by a nurse. She kicked vigorously, as she had been practicing for the past six weeks, and seemed to respond normally. The other babies were sleeping in bassinets near the window. Another visitor identified me as the new father, and pointed out Shirley Jane back by the sink as the new baby who had just come in.

164

My wife was pretty groggy still from the anesthetic and seemed quite disappointed that she couldn't carry the whole project off without sedation. But by Sunday morning, when she had had a good night's sleep, she walked down the corridor to the nursery to see our daughter. Although she was still stiff and sore, she seemed to be immensely cheerful. The one particular reaction she had in the recovery room was surprise that she could again see past her tummy.

In spite of the fact that she had to have sedation for the actual delivery and was out for two hours, the Lamaze training had two quite positive advantages. One was that she could stay in control of her contractions, which were very strong, for quite a long time. The other, possibly much more important in the long run, was that we both knew what to expect, and there was something relevant that I could do to help her with much of her labor period, from 8:30 in the morning, to the hospital at 1:30, until 5:30 when she finally went to sleep. It wasn't mysterious and scary—it just became very very painful.

We're both extremely happy with the outcome.

Sincerely,

Bob B.

John

DEAR MRS. BING:

After talking to you this morning, I began thinking back over my labor and delivery and realized that I remembered a lot of it. I wrote it down, and here it is:

The membranes broke at 8:30 P.M.—just as I had served up a splendid dinner of chili and salad and beer. So, remembering that one shouldn't eat after the labor starts, I sat ruefully watching my husband eat and had a comforting beer myself. Several hours went by and nothing happened. Nothing, except more water; how could there be so much water, and what if I hadn't been home when it happened? I decided to get some sleep, and my husband and I lay down for an hour's nap—though it really wasn't much of a nap, because we were so excited. Finally, the labor seemed to start in earnest, and when contractions were four minutes apart we called the doctor, who said to come to the hospital. By this time we were wildly excited and nervous too, though we joked ferociously as we drove through town at 2:30 in the morning. The people at the hospital desk were all very jolly as we checked in. "Oh, it's full moon tonight," they said. "There's always a lot of babies with full moon." And so there seemed to be.

We settled into the labor room and everything seemed

166

to be fine. I was in what appeared to be the accelerated part of the first stage of labor, the doctor was pleased and went off to sleep on a cot nearby, and I had a lollipop. Then everything came to a halt and labor stopped. The doctor was summoned and decided to give me oral doses of pitocin to start things off again. The contractions became more frequent again and much stronger, but on examination I still did not dilate any further. The head nurse came by and told me that if I persisted in this exaggerated breathing (which seemed absolutely necessary from my point of view) I would exhaust myself by the time the delivery actually occurred. Her advice was to practice self-control. I was getting exhausted, but self-control was not really one of the exercises, and I wasn't prepared for it. I spent a miserable couple of hours; I was sure I had failed already —and then, suddenly, on the next examination, I apparently had made good progress with dilation.

Even so, I began to consider giving up. It seemed impossible to go on; it was 10 A.M. by now, and the doctor had said that it might take till 2 P.M. for the baby to arrive. Why am I doing this? I kept wondering; because I paid to go to the classes and dragged my husband to them and I want it to be worth all that effort? At that point I didn't know why, and I couldn't think of a good reason.

Then suddenly I remembered that the grumpiness and the feeling that you just couldn't take any more were signs that you were nearly ready to deliver.

"Wake up the doctor," I said brightly. "I think I'm ready to deliver!" The nurses were sweet. "Oh, no, dear, he was just here and you were only eight and a half cm dilated, we really can't disturb him for another check so soon." "All right," I said, remembering that the doctor had to approve my medication, "I'd like to be sedated."

So the doctor came and was equally doubtful, but I was feeling more and more like pushing and could hardly stop myself. "O.K.," he said, "go ahead and push." It felt great. He looked again and said, "Now, here we go, we haven't much time left." I was ecstatic; the baby was really coming now, and suddenly I had all the energy in the world. My husband's mask and gown were checked and I was moved from the bed to the delivery room.

Then the real pushing began. After two good pushes the doctor said, "Now I'm going to ask you not to push for a while." I agreed, and panted and blew, but then suddenly there the baby was—there was a quick and painless episiotomy, one last big push and there was his head. It was a glorious push, the most satisfying thing in the world. And then he howled. "What is it?" I asked, though I could perfectly well see that he wasn't entirely born yet. "Just a minute," the doctor said, but he was getting excited too. Another push and a gigantic boy wriggled out and howled again, his mouth open enormously like a cobra's. The sound was almost a quack. "It's a duck!" my husband yelled, and I kept thinking, Oh, dear, we are both going to cry, as we had at all the birth movies, and we did. But everyone was excited; I thought the staff would be bored and uninterested, but they seemed almost as jubilant as we were. The doctor explained that they had not seen many Lamaze births and they always found them fascinating. Everyone was very pleased that he was such a big (nine pounds, one and a half ounces) well-formed baby, and the doctor promptly pronounced me one of his two best deliverers—when only a few hours earlier I had been convinced of my failure.

Then the repair of the episiotomy, which seemed anticlimactic; I wanted to see my baby and talk to my husband, my excitement was running so high. In fact, I didn't sleep for a week despite sleeping pills, and my husband didn't either.

I've never been so overwhelmed by emotion or so excited. If I hadn't known before why I was taking the course and trying the Lamaze method, I certainly knew now. I couldn't possibly have imagined the depth of the experience beforehand, and looking back, I can't imagine that anything else in my life will equal it.

Sincerely,
FRAN M.

Benjamin

••

DEAR MRS. BING:

On the Monday previous to our delivery I was admitted
to the hospital for treatment of phlebitis. By Thursday
I had developed what they thought then to be a kidney
infection. By Friday morning I was thoroughly discouraged. I had been up all night with horrible pain that began at the left kidney and literally wrapped itself around
me (breathing techniques didn't work). The doctor decided to induce labor. By then I didn't care what they
did to me—in fact, if they had wanted to do a section
I would not have been at all upset. At 8:30 A.M. my husband and I were in the labor room. All I had to do was
to see the IV glucose and pitocin, which would have tied
up my arms . . . I decided this was not for me, and proceeded to go into nice hard labor on my own!

We realized that I was having contractions that were
lasting up to seventy seconds with an interval of three
minutes—and when this became a real pattern my entire
attitude changed, and we went to work! The interesting
thing was that I had had no sleep and had been given
a sleeping pill off and on during the night, yet I felt as
though I had slept an entire night and woken up to a
beautiful morning. The doctor broke my membranes, and

as my husband watched the water pouring out he said, "It looks like Tinicum Creek," to which the doctor replied, "Yes, but there are no tin cans!"

By 11:30 A.M. I was 6 cm dilated. We were working very hard, but staying on top and relaxing extremely well between contractions. I can't say how important the relaxation exercises were—during transition, which was extremely difficult, I was like a rag doll.

At noon the hospital offered my husband a hot lunch, which he ate in the doctors' room. At this time a lovely nurse stayed with me and gave me encouragement.

By 1:30 P.M. I had the urge to push, but was only 8 cm dilated, and here is where we forgot our training. The nurse said that I should try pushing to see if the head was coming down, and instead of doing it correctly I not only forgot to pull my legs up but was pushing with my throat . . . we think that if I had done this correctly we would have cut a lot of time. At this point I was very tired since I was constantly blowing out and having only thirty seconds between contractions that lasted to almost three minutes. I was given 50 mg of Demerol, which took the edge off and allowed me to rest between contractions. The last two hours were hard, and if it hadn't been for my husband I would not have made it. I'm sure that two things saved the day: one was that I was in excellent physical condition (in spite of the kidney trouble), and another is that I don't smoke, for I was blowing out for two to three minutes at a time and was not getting winded. When I would start to lose control, my husband was there to put me back on the track by either giving me commands or breathing with me. Although I didn't feel like rubbing my stomach at this point, my husband did it, and this felt very good.

Finally, the delivery room! I was told not to push while the sterile leggings were put on me and an antiseptic was poured between my legs, which felt divine, and I was given a shot of Novocain for the episiotomy—and then I was allowed to push. It was the greatest feeling to be able to push. There was absolutely no pain, only immense excitement to see our baby—and lo and behold, before I knew it, they were all yelling for me to look down away from the mirror to see our baby coming for real . . . and after all those years of wishing and waiting there he was, all 8 pounds 14 ounces of Benjamin. I honestly cannot describe in words how I felt. All I remember saying is "I love you, darling" and "How beautiful, how beautiful!" My husband said that he wished he had had a tape recorder for the sounds I made, which told the whole story. The stitching took about thirty minutes and was the most uncomfortable part of it all, but I was relaxed and excited and didn't mind. An hour later, Benjamin was nursing and my husband was next to me and we were on the telephone letting everyone hear Benjamin coo.

A couple of days later I met a woman who had her baby the same day, and she asked if I was the one in the delivery room screaming at the top of my lungs, and when I told her no, she said that she was sure I must have been the one that sounded as if she was a locomotive pulling into the station! And pull into the station we did with our horn tooting and Benjamin in the caboose!

Sincerely,
MICHELLE G.

Peter

●━━━━━━━━━━━━━━━━━━━━━━━━━━━━━━━━●

DEAR MRS. BING:

This is a brief, belated "father's report" on the birth of our son on March 11 by the Lamaze method. I have tried to combine some personal reactions and the sequence of events, which was difficult to do. However, here it is:

My wife and I were introduced to the Lamaze method by friends, two couples who had had success with it and had expressed their enthusiasm for it to us. At first we were not convinced that we would follow through with it during the actual birth of our child, but we attended the classes with two objectives:

1. To help us anticipate the sequence of events in childbirth so that we could cope with the process intelligently; and

2. To gain skills which would make the day of labor more comfortable for her, even if we did not follow the method through to the end.

As it turned out, we became quite enthused with the method, and we followed through with it entirely in the birth process. Upon reflection afterward, we discovered one other equally important, perhaps more important, reason for which we would do it over again and commend the method to others. That means that in this method there is a built-in human factor. The wife is in control of her emotions, and—because husband and wife work together—the couple find that they are treated as participants in the birth of their child. In every case our questions were answered. In every case, after the doctor's examination, he summoned me back to the labor room and told me about her condition and what to expect. The nurse was very helpful. She kept us informed of progress, answered questions, and frequently gave words of encouragement. This was a far cry from what went on in nearby labor rooms. There we heard shrieks from women who were "knocked out," and the response of hospital personnel to them consisted of remarks such as, "Oh, hush! You're not so bad off."

We are pleased with the success of the birth. All went well even though this was our first child (first labors are usually more difficult than subsequent ones); also, the baby was large—eight pounds, ten ounces—and my wife's labor was not of the textbook variety.

Her labor began sometime after 6:30 P.M. on Monday night. At 8:50 P.M., after the dishes were washed and put away, we decided to start clocking contractions. We timed them until 9:30 and, surprisingly, they were coming every five minutes or less. We called the doctor, but he wasn't immediately available. By the time he got back to us it was 9:45 P.M. He told us to "start thinking about coming to the hospital." We got there at 10:10 P.M. By midnight, after prepping, my wife was in the labor room. Her contractions came very rapidly—one immediately after the other at times. They seemed to come in pairs. At 1:15 A.M. the doctor checked her, and she was at 4 cm dilation. Now the contractions came even more rapidly and more intensely. Still on top of her situation, however, she used the accelerated breathing technique. It was about all she could handle, but she kept with it successfully. At 1:35 A.M. she had an injection of Demerol. This helped her relax between contractions. It was 2:15 A.M. when she had the urge to push. My first reaction was, No, that's impossible; she had been only 4 cm at 1:15! But the doctor checked her, and much to the surprise of both my wife and me, she was now fully dilated and could push. She found that pushing was a great relief. Since the child was large, and our first, the pushing lasted for a long time— nearly two hours. At 4:06 A.M. our son Peter was born. What an amazing event to see him enter the world, to begin breathing, open his eyes, and wail softly from time to time.

There are the more personal memories of the night— both humorous and dramatic—which cannot be expressed here, but shall be remembered with pleasure.

Thank you again for your instruction and your interest.

Sincerely,

ARTHUR H.

Joshua

●●

Dear Mrs. Bing:

We were lucky enough to have had our first baby in
France. Though the circumstances were hectic, and though
my training was not very adequate, still the actual delivery was an enormous thrill to my husband and me: I had
no medication, and I had at least learned to push with
real effectiveness. The birth of our daughter was such a
joy to us both that we wanted, of course, to repeat the
experience with the coming of our second baby.

This time, however, we were living in Tennessee. After
combing out the area we found, disappointingly, that no
hospital in the region would permit a husband in the
delivery room ("hospital policy," which the more honest
doctors admitted is only made by doctors themselves).

We therefore decided to go to New York (my home
town) to have our baby. We shopped by mail for a doctor and were exceedingly delighted with our choice. My
husband arranged to work in a lab in New York during
our stay. My parents were able to house us all. Two very
doting grandparents would help look after our daughter,
so the only thing that remained was to find baby sitters
for our tropical fish and to become letter-perfect in our
Lamaze technique.

By some fluke, I had come across a copy of *Six Prac-*

176

tical Lessons for an Easier Childbirth. Lucky for me, I snatched it up, because I don't think another copy has been seen in the town since. We applied ourselves to it religiously (my husband says I was horribly compulsive), but I guess I felt I could hardly drag my whole family to New York—and just the whole nerve of it all—and not come through with "my stuff" in the end.

We arrived in New York three weeks before my due date. We had a "refresher" session with you and we received tremendous moral support when we found out that we had indeed been practicing correctly all along. And we also received some very specific and invaluable pointers which helped me during labor, such as the two tennis balls for back labor or backache. They aroused the nurses' amused curiosity, but they certainly helped when I had backache during labor. Other points underlined in this session were: to sit up and not to lie down flat during labor. (I sat comfortably in a chair up to 5 cm dilation and then moved to a raised bed. Then it was greatly impressed upon me that one simply must not push until given permission by the doctor. I had read various suggestions about what to do in order not to push when you feel the urge: one book said "pant-blow," my doctor said to pant—but you had said that if the urge is at all strong, blowing out continuously would be the most effective way. During transition and expulsion I found that you were very right. And when I asked my doctor, he said, "I don't care what you do, as long as you don't push!"

By the middle of the last week before my due date, I was effaced and 2 cm dilated; so we decided for convenience that I would be induced a couple of days early, if the baby didn't arrive on his own by then.

We began the great day by gorging ourselves on a huge early breakfast (I was going to need lots of energy for labor, and the bacon and eggs would all be digested by the time labor would start). The pitocin drip was begun at 10 A.M. and the doctor predicted that we'd have a baby by 2 or 2:30 P.M. Until 1:30 P.M. I sat in a chair reading and kidding my husband as we looked together without success at a list of 100,000 girls' names (we were sure that Eve was going to have a sister). Though nothing much was happening, the time flew, and I know that was because my husband was with me. From noon or thereabouts I felt mild contractions, like rather strong menstrual cramps, but there was no need to do any special breathing. I finished one book and began another, and the doctor said I still looked too happy for anything much to be happening.

At 1:30 P.M. I was 4 cm dilated. My husband went off for lunch; and by 2 P.M. I started special breathing, staying with the first breathing as long as possible. Then I switched to the rapid breathing, and I found to my surprise that once I got through the peak of each contraction I felt simply like stopping and exhaling slowly and sighing instead of finishing off with the slowing-down breaths which I'd practiced. (This was a very "physical" decision I made—not a cerebral one at all—as if my body was telling me that it would be more restful and energy-saving to breathe this way.)

My spirits were high. I was managing fine with the contractions, which were growing stronger. My husband was by my side—he gave me the full details of the hospital lunch menu—and I guess that was the last extraneous matter which we discussed.

My doctor broke my membranes, and then things moved faster than I'd ever dreamed. I switched automatically to pant-blow breathing, which worked wonderfully well for me. After a very strong contraction with mounting rectal pressure, I told my husband in no uncertain terms to get the doctor. He pronounced me 8 cm dilated. I heard the words "bloody show" and the wonderful word "transition." A rolling bed was gotten in haste, and by 3:25 P.M. I was on my way to the delivery room. En route, I demanded, "Push?" and the doctor said, "No, pant-blow."

Sterile leggings were hastily drawn on me. The doctor (bless his heart) made sure that pillows were propped under my back. My husband (bless his heart) made sure that my missing hand grip was found and replaced. I had two more extremely strong contractions when I could feel the baby pushing down . . . I had the feeling that everyone was dashing around with great urgency washing hands, and all I wanted to do was push! At this moment especially, my husband was my great anchor of calmness, telling me I was doing great, and just *looking* calm and somehow "proud papa" already. I soon was asking very urgently, "May I push?" A nurse listened to the fetal heart, and the doctor said, "Push!" and off I went in blissful relief. The head emerged in two pushes—the only work left to do was a bit more pushing and "stop pushing." Every time the doctor said "Stop," I blew out continuously and I found that I was indeed able to push and stop pushing on command. It was certainly a wonderful feeling to be that much on top of a stressful situation.

At the risk of sounding silly, I'll mention one other thing: From the training record and from our practicing, I'd somehow expected to sound utterly calm—panting in polite, ladylike fashion, even under the strongest fear of very active labor. Well, I made a bit more noise than that—I huffed and panted and blew loud and hard; but even while sounding like a raspy steam engine, I was always in complete control of my labor. It wouldn't have

179

occurred to me to scream, and it was simply a matter of chugging along till the end.

And what a marvelous "ending" to the story and to my work: the beginning of a whole new life of this glistening, wondrous, cuddly creature I pushed out of me into the afternoon light. I shall treasure forever the first sight of his first frown, the first sound of his first mewing cry. The pearly cord which attached him to me was lustrous—and I thought I'd burst for joy when I hugged my son for the first time, all warm and all ours now, on my flat belly.

I'll never forget the pride and excitement on my husband's face—and that look alone made me want to do it all over again right away. I just can't imagine doing Lamaze without my husband present: you can't chop up an experience which so obviously belongs to the three of you. (Of course, I also can't imagine my husband feeling any differently from the way he does about childbirth. But every now and then I stop and marvel at the trouble he went to to get us all in one piece to New York.)

I felt rapturous and ravenous and was free to gaze at our baby while I was cleaned up. Yes, I did experience pain, but it wasn't like some senseless toothache, it was always controllable and always purposeful. I always knew that there'd be a baby in the end!

But more than that, I wouldn't have wanted to deaden what pain there was, because that also would have numbed the intensity of my joy. I took part in the birth of our son with an utter completeness of body and feeling. We're lucky to have had Josh in this extraordinary, fine way, a way which worked like a charm for ordinary mortals like us.

Sincerely,
JUDY W.

Alexandra

DEAR MRS. BING:

It went "more or less by the book" and it went beautifully. Natural, or maybe "artificial" would be a better
word, childbirth, really works. I had a 5 pound, 14 ounce
flaxen-haired little girl, Alexandra, with a delicate, pretty
face and disposition to match.

It started the evening of October 9th. I had had an
examination by the doctor, who had told me that I was
ready to "pop," it was already three days past my due
date, and I was growing rather impatient, weary of not
being able to tie my shoelaces. At any rate, my husband
and I were busy painting and staining louvered doors; the
ground floor of our brownstone was in a state of uproar—
everywhere something had to be finished. While I was
putting the finishing touches of varnish on one of the
doors I felt mild cramps in my groin. I also noticed that
I was staining a little when I went to the bathroom, but
I figured that might be the result of my visit to the doctor. I called his office. The doctor was not in and the
operator of his answering service asked if I were actively
bleeding or just staining. I confessed to being a novice
and said I didn't know. She promised to notify the doctor, and, comforted, I returned to my doors. When the
doctor called back I was having mild cramps—from eight

to eleven minutes apart. He reassured me that he was right by the phone, and said that I should wait till the contractions came six to seven minutes apart and then call him.

I was feeling rather tired, exhausted, in fact, as I had been feeling all day. So at 11:30 my husband and I went to sleep. I was frankly hoping nothing would happen till the morning, since I was so overwhelmingly sleepy. At 2 A.M. I woke with more intense cramps than before. I timed them about seven minutes apart. After half an hour I woke Rob, we timed the contractions together for a while, then called the doctor. He told us to get to the hospital. We were very calm; we didn't even rush around. Rob had gotten a sandwich and beer earlier in the evening; we packed our Lamaze bag, including the lollipops, and called a cab.

We were so calm and jokey on the way to the hospital that we upset the driver. He felt we should be more flustered. I wore a pair of sneakers and slacks. I must have looked like I was going on a camping trip. When we got to the hospital, another of my doctor's patients was also being admitted. I had seen her in the waiting room a few times. We were taken to the same prep room, and as we were both candidates for the Lamaze method, we struck up an instant comradeship. We laughed and joked through the curtain. This was the other lady's third child. I felt as though it were my third child too.

After I had been questioned and prepped, the resident, an extremely pleasant man, examined me internally and pronounced me 4 to 5 cm dilated already. He also commented on the fact that I seemed so relaxed and happy. I was encouraged by the progress I had made before coming to the hospital. I was doing the first-phase breathing while I was prepped. I massaged the groin, back and forth; it was very soothing. I felt as though I were going to be able to control my physical reactions.

By the time I got to the labor room it was 5 A.M. My husband was called, and I used the deep breathing for a while. I had the bed partially cranked up. Rob was encouraging me to relax, testing my arms and legs during contractions to see if I was. He was wonderfully helpful, putting the washcloth in my mouth, testing my degree of relaxation, sprinkling powder on my abdomen. Many times during labor he put his arm under my head. Just having him physically close to me was beautiful.

The nurse brought in the heartbeat amplifier, and Rob heard the beating of the baby's heart underwater, as it were. The membranes had not been broken. In fact, they did not break until I was on the delivery table. The contractions were coming about three minutes apart after about three hours in the labor room. I then used the second phase breathing, and pretty successfully too. I found it very easy, much easier than when I had practiced it at home. It came very naturally. But then I was 8 cm dilated and things started getting rough. The contractions shot up like firecrackers, with me, at times, in breathless pursuit. I started the pant-blow breathing, but it took all my concentration not to cry out, the contractions were so forceful. My husband kept on saying "Relax, Joan!" and I could see my toes curling up involuntarily. By this time my husband's verbal suggestions were getting irritating— but I was still polite! I *requested* that he not speak to me any more during a contraction.

By this time I was experiencing the urge to push—like an overwhelming desire to move my bowels—which rapidly shifted to a more abdominal sensation. I caught it by blowing right from the start of a contraction, with but the cleansing breath at the very beginning.

By that time there were about six nurses in the room, including two wide-eyed student nurses who had never seen a Lamaze childbirth before. One of the nurses immediately told me to concentrate, keep my eyes open and keep breathing regularly. She obviously knew the Lamaze technique very well. However, I could not keep my eyes open at this point. My doctor came in and asked me whether I wanted a little Demerol so I could relax better between contractions. I agreed because I was having trouble relaxing at this point. The Demerol did relax me enough that I could stay in control, and very soon I was told that I could start to push.

I grabbed the siderails, took a couple of deep breaths and pushed. Everyone was encouraging me. "You are doing wonderfully!" "Two more pushes," my doctor said, "and the head will be out!" I was trying to push as hard as I could with each contraction, but it seemed very hard. However, something must have been happening, because I was suddenly taken on a stretcher to the delivery room.

In the delivery room, of course, everything was done with incredible speed. My husband was there, standing to one side. I was urged to push, which I did, but it felt as if the head was stuck. The anesthesiologist asked me whether I wanted a little gas to help me push. She stuck the mask over my nose, but I was trying so hard to hold my breath and push that I was unable to breathe much of the gas in. Then suddenly the membranes broke, and the baby's head and body just popped out (according to Rob). She cried a little as soon as she emerged, then she was cleaned up. She was held up to me as soon as she came out and I was told she was a girl. I remember saying with disbelief, "Is there really a baby?" I don't think I ever believed there really was a live creature in there. My husband bent over and kissed me, and I saw the doctor shake his hand and congratulate him.

The crowd of nurses disappeared, leaving the two student nurses. They were both ga-ga about the whole experience. They were both enormously impressed with this childbirth method, and particularly with the way my husband and I had been with each other and given birth together. "It was beautiful," they said, and I felt very gratified.

I was taken to the rooming-in ward and I saw my baby after a while. I spent some time with my husband, who was so happy he was ready to burst, and then I fell asleep for a while.

In summary: The experience was thrilling, uplifting, immensely satisfying and aesthetic. I will do it willingly again. There was considerable pain at the end, but it was bearable, and I struggled with it. The Demerol at the end helped me relax. I was awake and aware, and I felt emotionally everything there was to feel, feelings that make psychoprophylaxis such a marvelous method to use in labor and delivery.

Sincerely,
JOAN Y.

EDITOR'S NOTE:

One of the most important aspects of a prepared labor is that the young woman trusts her physician, and that she feels assured that he is on her side. In many cases labor becomes almost overwhelmingly strong toward the end of the first stage. It is then that the physician's encouragement or his advice to take a little sedation to help relaxation is so important and should be accepted by the mother. Being helped during a difficult stretch does not mean "failure." It only means that there should be teamwork between parents and physician, trust on both sides and encouragement. It never makes sense to hold out and refuse help, when help can be the means to be actively participating in the birth of the child.

Joan certainly feels that her experience was a very positive one, even if she needed medication to help her for a while.

Epilogue

I tried from time to time in this little volume to explain or discuss the individual report. However, after a short while, I realized that there was very little I could add to the parents' accounts. Surely they speak for themselves.

One of my students asked the other day to bring her mother to the class, as her husband was unable to come. The mother, a most attractive woman, sat through the class spellbound, it seemed to me. She never said anything during the session, but when I occasionally glanced at her I saw her watching her daughter closely as we were practicing the Lamaze technique, and she was also watching all the other couples with obvious interest. When the lesson was over, the mother smiled at the group, saying, "You know, I have had four children, and by the time I had my fourth I did not know as much about labor and delivery as you people seem to know now, expecting your first child. I had to learn what to do with each labor and delivery, and there was nobody who ever told me what to do." And then she added, "You are so lucky, I envy you!"

I grinned and nodded, agreeing with her wholeheartedly, and I also suddenly remembered my own mother, who years ago watched one of my classes, getting up spontaneously after the class and saying, "I've had five children, and I wish someone had taught me how to handle my labors."

And a few weeks ago, I called one of the obstetricians, who had sent me a number of his patients, to discuss a medical matter with him and also to thank him for referring patients to me. "Oh, well," he answered, "I love to send the girls, it's so much more fun for me to help a woman in labor who is lucid, whom I can communicate with, and who has such confidence in herself and her ability to perform a difficult job. I enjoy my work this way."

Childbirth is a supreme experience in life for most of us, and if we can make it a rewarding experience and enjoyable and medically safe at the same time, the opportunity to achieve this should be available for every woman and her husband.

As this is an epilogue, I want to end the book on a very personal note and say "Thank you, thank you" to all my students for being such interested and lively students; for helping all of us who teach the Lamaze method to feel that we are doing a worthwhile job; and finally for persuading their own friends that childbirth can be a joyful experience.

Bibliography

Bing, Elisabeth D., R.P.T., *Six Practical Lessons for an Easier Childbirth*. New York, A Rutledge Book, Grosset & Dunlap, 1967.

Bing, Elisabeth D., R.P.T., Karmel, Marjorie, and Tanz, Alfred, M. D., *A Practical Training Course for the Psychoprophylactic Method of Childbirth (Lamaze Technique)*, Fifth Printing, New York, A.S.P.O, 36 West 96 Street, New York, N.Y. 10025.

Bonstein, Isidore, M.D., *Psychoprophylactic Preparation for Painless Childbirth*. New York, Grune & Stratton, Inc., 1958.

Chabon, Irwin, M.D., *Awake and Aware: Participating in Childbirth through Prophylaxis*. New York, Delacorte Press, 1966. Paperback, New York, Dell Publishing Company, Inc., 1969.

Flanagan, Geraldine Lux, *The First Nine Months of Life*. New York, Simon and Schuster, 1962.

Karmel, Marjorie, *Thank You, Dr. Lamaze*. Philadelphia, J. B. Lippincott, 1959. Paperback, Garden City, New York, Dolphin Books, Doubleday & Co., Inc., 1965.

Rennert, Zila, M.D., *L'Enseignement de l'accouchement sans douleur: Comment le préparer et le diriger gymnastique pré et postnatale*. Paris, Vigot Frères, Éditeurs, 23 rue de l'École-de-Médicine.

Vellay, Pierre, M.D., *Childbirth with Confidence*. New York, Macmillan Co., 1969.

189

Vellay, Pierre, M.D., and Others, *Childbirth Without Pain.* New York, E. P. Dutton & Co., Inc., 1959.

Velvovsky, I., Platonov, K., Ploticher, V., Shugom, E., *Painless Childbirth Through Psychoprophylaxis* (*Lectures for Obstetricians*). Moscow, Foreign Languages Publishing House, 1960.

For further information, contact:

The American Society for Psychoprophylaxis in Obstetrics, Inc., 36 West 96th Street, New York, N.Y., 10025

Glossary

Analgesia   Pain relief

Anesthesia   Insensibility (no consciousness)

Bag of waters   Membrane enclosing the fluid around the fetus

Bloody show   A discharge of mucus tinged with blood; frequently occurs just prior to onset of labor

Braxton-Hicks contractions   Intermittent, painless contractions of the uterus toward the end of pregnancy

Breech birth   The presenting part of the baby is the buttocks or one or both feet

Caesarean section   Removal of the baby by incision through the abdominal wall and uterus

Cervix   Neck of womb

Cleansing breath   A deep, relaxing inhalation-exhalation to be taken at the beginning and end of each contraction

Demerol   An analgesic (pain reliever) frequently administered in labor to aid relaxation

Dilatation (dilation) of cervix   Opening of cervix to 10 cm or five fingers

Effacement of cervix   Thinning out and flattening of the neck of the uterus

Episiotomy   Small incision into perineum to prevent tearing during birth of baby

Goody bag   A small bag to hold washcloth, powder, picture (to focus on), lollipops, chapstick, etc.

Karmel, Marjorie   Author of *Thank you, Dr. Lamaze*, the book which was most instrumental in introducing the Lamaze technique into the United States

Paracervical block   A regional anesthetic which blocks the pain sensation during the dilatation of the cervix

Partial prep   Clipping of pubic hair only (in contrast to a "full prep" where pubic and pelvic floor hair is shaved)

Pitocin   A hormone, given either intravenously or in the form of a small flat pill placed under the lip, to induce or speed up labor

Placenta   Afterbirth

Sphincter exercises   Contracting and relaxing the urinary and rectal openings, as well as tightening and relaxing the vagina (also called Kegel exercises)

Transition   The last 2–3 cm of dilatation of the cervix, before pushing